Advances in Obstetric Ultrasound

Guest Editors

THEODORE J. DUBINSKY, MD
MANJIRI DIGHE, MD

ULTRASOUND CLINICS

www.ultrasound.theclinics.com

Consulting Editor
VIKRAM S. DOGRA, MD

January 2011 • Volume 6 • Number 1

SAUNDERS an imprint of ELSEVIER, Inc.

W.B. SAUNDERS COMPANY
A Division of Elsevier Inc.

1600 John F. Kennedy Boulevard • Suite 1800 • Philadelphia, Pennsylvania 19103-2899

http://www.theclinics.com

ULTRASOUND CLINICS Volume 6, Number 1
January 2011 ISSN 1556-858X, ISBN-13: 978-1-4557-0514-6

Editor: Barton Dudlick

Ultrasound Clinics (ISSN 1556-858X) is published quarterly by W.B. Saunders, 360 Park Avenue South, New York, NY 10010-1710. Months of publication are January, April, July, and October. Business and editorial offices: 1600 John F. Kennedy Boulevard, Suite 1800, Philadelphia, Pennsylvania 19103-2899. Accounting and circulation offices: 6277 Sea Harbor Drive, Orlando, FL 32887-4800. Periodicals postage paid at New York, NY, and additional mailing offices. Subscription prices are $225 per year for (US individuals), $279 per year for (US institutions), $107 per year for (US students and residents), $253 per year for (Canadian individuals), $312 per year for (Canadian institutions), $269 per year for (international individuals), $312 per year for (international institutions), and $129 per year for (Canadian and foreign students/residents). To receive student/resident rate, orders must be accompanied by name of affiliated institution, date of term, and the signature of program/residency coordinator on institution letterhead. Orders will be billed at individual rate until proof of status is received. Foreign air speed delivery is included in all Clinics subscription prices. All prices are subject to change without notice. **POSTMASTER:** Send address changes to *Ultrasound Clinics,* Elsevier Health Sciences Division, Subscription Customer Service, 3251 Riverport Lane, Maryland Heights, MO 63043. **Customer Service (orders, claims, online, change of address): Telephone: 1-800-654-2452 (U.S. and Canada); 314-447-8871 (outside U.S. and Canada). Fax: 314-447-8029. E-mail: journalscustomerservice-usa@elsevier.com (for print support); journalsonlinesupport-usa@elsevier.com (for online support).**

Reprints: For copies of 100 or more, of articles in this publication, please contact the Commercial Reprints Department, Elsevier Inc., 360 Park Avenue South, New York, NY 10010-1710. Tel.: (+1) 212-633-3812; Fax: (+1) 212-462-1935; E-mail: reprints@elsevier.com.

Printed and bound by CPI Group (UK) Ltd, Croydon, CR0 4YY

Transferred to Digital Print 2011

Contributors

CONSULTING EDITOR

VIKRAM S. DOGRA, MD
Professor of Radiology, Urology, and
Biomedical Engineering; Director of Ultrasound
and Associate Chair for Education and
Research, Department of Imaging Sciences,
University of Rochester School of Medicine
and Dentistry, Rochester, New York

GUEST EDITORS

THEODORE J. DUBINSKY, MD
Laurence A. Mack Endowed Professor
of Radiology, Obstetrics, and Gynecology,
and Reproductive Health Sciences,
University of Washington, Seattle,
Washington

MANJIRI DIGHE, MD
Assistant Professor, Radiology Body Imaging,
University School of Medicine; Director of
Ultrasound, University of Washington Medical
Center, Seattle, Washington

AUTHORS

PUNEET BHARGAVA, MBBS, DNB
Assistant Professor, Department of Radiology,
University of Washington; Staff Radiologist,
Diagnostic Imaging Services, Veterans Affairs
Puget Sound Health Care System, Seattle,
Washington

MICHELLE BITTLE, MD
Harborview Medical Center, Department
of Radiology, Seattle, Washington

EDITH Y. CHENG, MD, MS
Professor, Division of Maternal Fetal Medicine,
Department of Obstetrics and Gynecology;
Adjunct Associate Professor, Division of
Medical Genetics, Department of Internal
Medicine, University of Washington, Seattle,
Washington

CARLOS CUEVAS, MD
Assistant Professor, Department of
Radiology, University of Washington,
Seattle, Washington

MANJIRI DIGHE, MD
Associate Professor of Radiology, University
of Washington; Director of Body Imaging,
Seattle, Washington

THEODORE J. DUBINSKY, MD
Laurence A. Mack Endowed Professor
of Radiology Obstetrics and Gynecology,
and Reproductive Health Sciences University
of Washington, Seattle, Washington

CORINNE L. FLIGNER, MD
Associate Professor, Pathology; Adjunct
Associate Professor, Laboratory Medicine,
Anatomic Pathology; Director, Autopsy and
After Death Services, University of Washington
School of Medicine, University of Washington
Medical Center, Seattle, Washington

MARK B. LEWIN, MD
Associate Professor of Pediatrics; Chief,
Division of Cardiology, Seattle Children's
Hospital, University of Washington School
of Medicine, Seattle, Washington

MARIAM MOSHIRI, MD
Clinical Assistant Professor, Director Body
Imaging Fellowship, Department of Radiology,
University of Washington Medical Center,
University of Washington School of Medicine,
Seattle, Washington

KATHY O'CONNELL, MN, RN
Department of Obstetrics and Gynecology,
University of Washington Medical Center,
Seattle, Washington

SOPHIA ROTHBERGER, MD
Senior Fellow, Maternal Fetal Medicine,
Obstetrics and Gynecology, University
of Washington School of Medicine, Seattle,
Washington

CLAUDIA SADRO, MD
Harborview Medical Center, Department
of Radiology, Seattle, Washington

A. LUANA STANESCU, MD
Instructor, Department of Radiology, Seattle
Children's Hospital, Seattle, Washington

MARGARET M. VERNON, MD
Assistant Professor of Pediatrics, Division
of Cardiology, Seattle Children's Hospital,
University of Washington School of Medicine,
Seattle, Washington

SARAH A. WALLER, MD
Clinical Instructor, Division of Obstetrics and
Gynecology, University of Washington, School
of Medicine, Seattle, Washington

Contents

> Currently, many screening options are available for evaluation of the genetic health of the fetus, with screening choices for Down syndrome that are complex in risk and benefit estimations. Health care providers have the responsibility of providing adequate counseling, access, and the most robust screening choices for patients. Comparative analyses of the various screening options to women interested in prenatal diagnosis indicate that at the screen positive rate of 5%, all screening approaches have high detection rates and can be offered to patients based on the availability of resources in the community and the gestational age during prenatal care.

> Techniques in ultrasonography have improved dramatically over the last several years. Ultrasonography provides patients with an excellent means of screening for anomalies, and the use of soft markers has individualized each patient's decision to pursue diagnostic testing. Consensus across disciplines, including radiology and obstetrics, is that a combined modality of maternal age, serum screening, and ultrasonography provides patients the best risk assessment. In the second trimester a normal ultrasonogram reduces the risk of trisomy 21 by 60% to 70% (likelihood ratio of 0.3–0.4) but does not completely negate it.

> A broad spectrum of orofacial anomalies can be detected by ultrasound. Awareness of their features can assist in diagnosis. Orofacial anomalies may be associated with other malformations, so additional studies may be needed to provide appropriate counseling information. Routine scanning of the fetal face in different planes by two-dimensional ultrasound during the second trimester provides most of the information needed. In addition, recent three-dimensional techniques allow for imaging of the fetal face with particular applicability to the evaluation of orofacial clefts. This article summarizes the features of orofacial anomalies detectable by ultrasound and the imaging techniques useful for early diagnosis.

> The selective use of complementary imaging modalities can significantly improve the detection and characterization of skeletal anomalies in the fetus. Three-dimensional ultrasonography can be used in a wide range of anatomic abnormalities, and seems to provide a significant advantage over 2-dimensional ultrasonography

for the study of fetal hands and feet. The use of computed tomography should be considered for the analysis of skeletal dysplasias, where it can provide extraordinarily good quality images of the entire skeleton. Magnetic resonance imaging is a safe modality that can provide useful additional information for complex fetal syndromes that involve multiple organ systems.

to a nonpregnant trauma patient, with radiography, computed tomography, and angiography to evaluate maternal injuries. In the major trauma patient, ultrasound is limited to fast scans in unstable patients and to evaluate the viability of the pregnancy. The most sensitive approach for diagnosing placental abruption is external fetal monitoring. Abnormal fetal heart tones are an indication for emergency cesarean delivery in cases of suspected placental abruption. Ultrasound is often performed to diagnose placental abruption but is falsely negative in 50–80% of cases.

Fetal/perinatal autopsy can identify the cause of demise, delineate abnormalities, and assist with establishing an etiology for malformations. Postmortem plain radiographs are a mainstay of skeletal abnormality evaluation. Postmortem MRI can sometimes provide structural detail of the CNS comparable to or better than traditional autopsy, but while useful in conjunction with limited or complete pathologic examination and ancillary diagnostic modalities, it does not have sufficient diagnostic accuracy to replace conventional autopsy at this time. Continued improvement in post-mortem diagnosis will require modification of MRI for postmortem use and small fetuses, development of novel tissue sampling modalities, and evaluation using well-designed, large, prospective studies.

Incidence of twinning is increasing, especially with the increase in the use of fertility treatment and advanced maternal age. Twin gestations cannot only have similar complications to sigelton pregnancies but at a higher rate, but also unique complications that are only seen in multiple gestations. The latter types of complications have variable presentations and are dependant on the type of twinning. Understanding the nature and appearance of these complications are of outmost importance in management of such pregnancies. This article discusses the imaging features of complications related to twin pregnancies.

There are situations in which competing goals for outcomes between the mother and the fetus compromise the mother to save the baby or generate permanent morbidity to the child to protect the mother's life. Abnormalities of placentation can cause significant maternal, fetal, and neonatal morbidity and mortality. Both ultrasonography and magnetic resonance imaging help in assessing the degree and location of placental invasion and in planning delivery. This article discusses 2 perinatal conditions that illustrate the complexity of the maternal and fetal relationship at delivery and the importance of multidisciplinary cooperation in enhancing successful outcomes for both mother and baby.

Ultrasound Clinics

THE CLINICS ARE NOW AVAILABLE ONLINE!

Access your subscription at:
www.theclinics.com

GOAL STATEMENT
The goal of the *Ultrasound Clinics* is to keep practicing radiologists and radiology residents up to date with current clinical practice in ultrasound by providing timely articles reviewing the state of the art in patient care.

ACCREDITATION
The *Ultrasound Clinics* is planned and implemented in accordance with the Essential Areas and Policies of the Accreditation Council for Continuing Medical Education (ACCME) through the joint sponsorship of the University of Virginia School of Medicine and Elsevier. The University of Virginia School of Medicine is accredited by the ACCME to provide continuing medical education for physicians.

The University of Virginia School of Medicine designates this educational activity for a maximum of 15 *AMA PRA Category 1 Credits*™ for each issue, 60 credits per year. Physicians should only claim credit commensurate with the extent of their participation in the activity.

The American Medical Association has determined that physicians not licensed in the US who participate in this CME activity are eligible for a maximum of 15 *AMA PRA Category 1 Credits*™ for each issue, 60 credits per year.

Credit can be earned by reading the text material, taking the CME examination online at http://www.theclinics.com/home/cme, and completing the evaluation. After taking the test, you will be required to review any and all incorrect answers. Following completion of the test and evaluation, your credit will be awarded and you may print your certificate.

FACULTY DISCLOSURE/CONFLICT OF INTEREST
The University of Virginia School of Medicine, as an ACCME accredited provider, endorses and strives to comply with the Accreditation Council for Continuing Medical Education (ACCME) Standards of Commercial Support, Commonwealth of Virginia statutes, University of Virginia policies and procedures, and associated federal and private regulations and guidelines on the need for disclosure and monitoring of proprietary and financial interests that may affect the scientific integrity and balance of content delivered in continuing medical education activities under our auspices.

The University of Virginia School of Medicine requires that all CME activities accredited through this institution be developed independently and be scientifically rigorous, balanced and objective in the presentation/discussion of its content, theories and practices.

All authors/editors participating in an accredited CME activity are expected to disclose to the readers relevant financial relationships with commercial entities occurring within the past 12 months (such as grants or research support, employee, consultant, stock holder, member of speakers bureau, etc.). The University of Virginia School of Medicine will employ appropriate mechanisms to resolve potential conflicts of interest to maintain the standards of fair and balanced education to the reader. Questions about specific strategies can be directed to the Office of Continuing Medical Education, University of Virginia School of Medicine, Charlottesville, Virginia.

The faculty and staff of the University of Virginia Office of Continuing Medical Education have no financial affiliations to disclose.

The authors/editors listed below have identified no professional or financial affiliations for themselves or their spouse/partner:
Puneet Bhargava, MBBS, DNB; Michelle Bittle, MD; Edith Y. Cheng, MD, MS; Manjiri Dighe, MD (Guest Editor); Theodore Dubinsky, MD (Guest Editor); Barton Dudlick, (Acquisitions Editor); Mark B. Lewin, MD; Mariam Moshiri, MD; Kathy O'Connell, MN, RN; Sophia Rothberger, MD; Claudia Sadro, MD; A. Luana Stanescu, MD; Margaret M. Vernon, MD; and Sarah A. Waller, MD.

The authors/editors listed below have identified the following professional or financial affiliations for themselves or their spouse/partner:
Matthew J. Bassignani, MD (Test Author) is on the Advisory Board/Committee for Nuance and Fuji Medical Systems.
Carlos Cuevas, MD is an industry funded research/investigator for Merck.
Vikram S. Dogra, MD (Consulting Editor) is the editor for the Journal of Clinical Imaging Science.
Corinne L. Fligner, MD's spouse is a consultant for Seattle Genetics and Amgen; is a speaker for Takeda Pharmaceutical; and is an industry funded researcher for BioRad and Dendreon.

Disclosure of Discussion of Non-FDA Approved Uses for Pharmaceutical Products and/or Medical Devices.
The University of Virginia School of Medicine, as an ACCME provider, requires that all faculty presenters identify and disclose any off-label uses for pharmaceutical and medical device products. The University of Virginia School of Medicine recommends that each physician fully review all the available data on new products or procedures prior to clinical use.

TO ENROLL
To enroll in the Ultrasound Clinics Continuing Medical Education program, call customer service at 1-800-654-2452 or visit us online at http://www.theclinics.com/home/cme. The CME program is available to subscribers for an additional fee of $196.00.

Preface
Advances in Obstetric Ultrasound

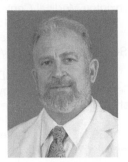 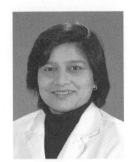

Theodore J. Dubinsky, MD   Manjiri Dighe, MD
Guest Editors

This issue of *Ultrasound Clinics* is dedicated to current advances in the imaging of both the fetus and the mother. Advances in ultrasound technology, MR, serology, and genetics have improved our ability to make sophisticated diagnoses in utero. In addition, advances in pathology have improved our understanding of fetal pathology as well. The development of the integrated screen for the detection of fetal chromosomal abnormalities has increased the sensitivity of prenatal diagnosis for Trisomy 21 to greater than 90%. This represents a significant advance compared to even 10 years ago when only 50% of Down's babies were detected prenatally.

The development of 3D ultrasound techniques has enhanced our ability to communicate with not only the referring obstetricians but the future caretakers of the fetus (ie, neonatalogists and pediatric surgeons) about the fetal abnormalities. This, in turn, has facilitated their ability to counsel patients and plan for the postnatal repair of these abnormalities. Applications of 3D ultrasound are relevant particularly to head and face imaging of the fetus, and for evaluation of musculoskeletal abnormalities. Advances in MR imaging, particularly the development of single breath-hold sequences and 3D sequences that minimize both fetal and maternal motion artifacts, have led to increased utilization of MR for fetal imaging. The ongoing realization that MR can depict pathology, particularly of the fetal CNS, and fetal neck masses and can add significant information about the prognosis and necessary treatment of a given fetal condition has led to an increased reliance on this modality for fetal abnormalities. Advances in the field of reproductive endocrinology and the incidence of multiple pregnancies have led to a greater need for specialized imaging like MRI. This is especially true in twin–twin transfusion and conjoined twins, where a great deal of anatomic information is necessary for delivery and surgical planning; both CT and MR have developed a greater role for evaluating twins subsequently. Disturbances of growth are as essential as ever to recognize and diagnose and are critical for delivery planning as well. Special circumstances can arise where maternal imaging is necessary such as in trauma or in maternal abdominal conditions, where

Ultrasound Clin 6 (2011) xi–xii
doi:10.1016/j.cult.2011.03.009

advances in CT technology have allowed faster scanning at reduced radiation exposure. These techniques have made CT quite reasonable and feasible in the appropriate circumstances. The development of new delivery strategies, especially the EXIT procedure, has created an increased demand for advanced in utero imaging to facilitate the planning for such deliveries as well as the care of the immediate postpartum neonate.

Ultimately, the quality assurance of a lab doing any sort of fetal imaging depends on the ability to get exquisite pathologic anatomic correlation and this improves our understanding of fetal development and hopefully improves our diagnostic capabilities as well. Hopefully, after reading this issue of *Ultrasound Clinics*, anyone performing any sort of imaging on a pregnant patient will gain insight and knowledge about the most current, state-of-the-art technology for evaluating

fetuses for the purposes of delivery planning, and postnatal therapy.

Theodore J. Dubinsky, MD
Department of Radiology
University of Washington Medical Center
Box 357115
1959 NE Pacific Street
Seattle, WA 98195, USA

Manjiri Dighe, MD
Department of Radiology
University of Washington Medical Center
Box 357115
1959 NE Pacific Street
Seattle, WA 98195, USA

E-mail addresses:
tdub@u.washington.edu (T.J. Dubinsky)
dighe@u.washington.edu (M. Dighe)

Prenatal Diagnosis: Noninvasive Screening

Edith Y. Cheng, MD, MS[a,b,*]

KEYWORDS

- Integrated screening • Nuchal translucency • Aneuploidy

Tremendous growth and expansion in the options for prenatal screening for birth defects and/or chromosome abnormalities have occurred in the past 40 years. The choices available today have been possible because of technological advancements in imaging and discoveries of associated biologic and biochemical changes in the abnormal fetus that could be detected through maternal serum screening and/or ultrasonography. In the late 1970s, 2 screening programs comprised the paradigms in prenatal diagnosis: elevated maternal serum α-fetoprotein (MSAFP) levels in the midtrimester for neural tube defects (NTD) and a maternal age of 35 years or more at delivery for Down syndrome. Both programs neither used imaging routinely as part of the prenatal screening process nor had high sensitivity for detecting the respective conditions. In 1984, biochemical screening for Down syndrome and trisomy 18 was introduced after Merkatz and colleagues[1] reported an association between low MSAFP levels and these 2 conditions. In the 1990s, human chorionic gonadotropin (hCG) and unconjugated estriol (UE$_3$) were added in the screening process, giving rise to the triple screen that improved the detection rate of Down syndrome and trisomy 18. Lastly, inhibin A was added to what is now known as the quadruple or quad screen, further improving the detection rate.[2] At the same time, major advances in ultrasonographic technology permitted earlier and clearer visualization of the fetus in the first trimester and of birth defects in the second trimester. Efforts directed at providing earlier prenatal screening and improved detection rates merged ultrasonography and maternal serum marker innovations to develop the integrated screen and its variants in the late 1990s. The First and Second Trimester Evaluation of Risk (FASTER) trial for fetal aneuploidy have since compared and demonstrated the efficacy of currently available prenatal screening approaches for Down syndrome prospectively in the general population.[3] In 2007, the American College of Obstetricians and Gynecologists recommended "… maternal age of 35 years alone should no longer be used as a cutoff to determine who is offered screening versus who is offered invasive testing."[4] **Fig. 1** summarizes the evolution of screening in prenatal diagnosis. This article discusses the principles of maternal prenatal screening and the current approaches to screening for Down syndrome.

MATERNAL SERUM SCREENING

The patterns of serum analyte levels for NTD, Down syndrome, and trisomy 18 and the detection rates using all current screening approaches are illustrated in **Tables 1** and **2**, respectively. Analyte levels are reported in multiples of median (MoM) to standardize the gestational age dependency of the interpretation of the levels. AFP is produced first in the fetal yolk sac and then in the fetal liver and serves essentially as the oncotic protein of the fetus. A break in the integrity of the fetal body, spine, abdominal wall, or skin is generally

[a] Division of Maternal Fetal Medicine, Department of Obstetrics and Gynecology, University of Washington, 1959 NE Pacific Street, Box 356460, Seattle, WA 98195, USA
[b] Division of Medical Genetics, Department of Internal Medicine, University of Washington, Seattle, WA, USA
* Division of Maternal Fetal Medicine, Department of Obstetrics and Gynecology, University of Washington, 1959 NE Pacific Street, Box 356460, Seattle, WA 98195.
E-mail address: chengels@u.washington.edu

Ultrasound Clin 6 (2011) 1–10
doi:10.1016/j.cult.2011.02.003

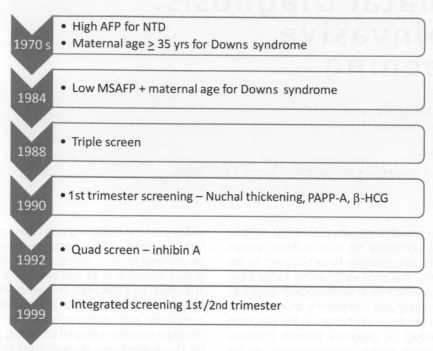

Fig. 1. Evolution of maternal serum screening strategies for NTD and Down syndrome in the last 40 years. In the 1970s, only a maternal age of 35 years or more at the time of delivery prompted Down syndrome screening, had a detection rate of 29%. MSAFP, maternal serum AFP; PAPP-A, pregnancy-associated plasma protein A.

associated with elevations of MSAFP levels in the amniotic fluid and maternal circulation. Before the routine use of imaging in pregnancy, an abnormal level of MSAFP was sometimes the first indication of a possible abnormality. A MSAFP level of 2.5 MoM or greater is used to identify pregnancies that need further evaluation. In combination with midtrimester imaging, the detection rate for open NTD is greater than 95%.[5] Definitive diagnosis is completed through midtrimester amniocentesis (15–22 weeks' gestation) for direct measurement of MSAFP levels in amniotic fluid, which should be elevated, and evaluation for the presence of acetylcholinesterase, which is specific for an open NTD. However, in conjunction with imaging, omphalocele, gastroschisis, and some inherited fetal dermatologic abnormalities are also detected. Elevated MSAFP levels are also associated with other fetal, maternal, and obstetric complications.[6]

The combination of low MSAFP and UE$_3$ levels and elevated total hCG and inhibin A levels forms the basis of the second-trimester (15–20 weeks' gestation) serum screening for Down syndrome. Individually, the analytes perform poorly in differentiating between affected and unaffected pregnancies. However, combining all 4 analytes together into a single screen provides a detection rate of about 81%, with a screen positive rate of 5%.[2,3] In fetuses with Down syndrome, the average MSAFP and UE$_3$ levels are 0.73 and 0.73 MoM, respectively[7]; the total hCG level is double of that of fetuses without Down syndrome at an average level of 2.06 MoM; and the inhibin A level is increased to 1.77 MoM.[2,8] In some second-trimester screening programs, the free β-hCG concentration is used because it seems to have a greater discriminatory value than total hCG levels; the average free β-hCG level is 2.66 MoM in fetuses with Down syndrome, which translates into a slightly higher detection rate.[7]

In trisomy 18, MSAFP, UE$_3$, and total hCG levels have a unique pattern in which levels of all 3 analytes are markedly decreased; the inhibin level is not measured because it does increase the discriminatory value of this analyte pattern for trisomy 18.[7] Likelihood ratios (LRs) are generated for each analyte based on a comparison of the proportion of affected pregnancies with a particular value with that of unaffected pregnancies with the same value. The final risk or adjusted risk (AR) is then a product of the patient's a priori risk (background risk [BR]) and the 4 LRs generated by the 4 analytes (AR = BR × LR). Implicit in this formula is the assumption that each analyte is an independent predictor of fetuses with Down

Table 1
Down syndrome screening tests and detection rates (5% screen positive rate)

Screening Test	Detection Rate (%)
First Trimester	
NT measurement	64–70
NT measurement, PAPP-A, free or total β-hCG[b]	82–87
Second Trimester	
Triple screen (MSAFP, hCG, UE₃)	69
Quadruple screen (MSAFP, hCG, UE₃, inhibin A)	81
First Plus Second Trimester	
Integrated (NT, PAPP-A quad screen)	94–96
Serum integrated (PAPP-A quad screen)	85–88

Stepwise sequential screen
First-trimester test result
   Positive: diagnostic test offered
   Negative: second-trimester test offered
   Final: risk assessment incorporates first and second results
	95

Contingent sequential screen First-trimester test result Positive: diagnostic test offered	88–94

Abbreviations: MSAFP, maternal serum AFP; NT, nuchal translucency; PAPP-A, pregnancy-associated plasma protein A.

From ACOG Committee on Practice Bulletins. ACOG Practice Bulletin No. 77: screening for fetal chromosomal abnormalities. Obstet Gynecol 2007;109:218; with permission.

syndrome. **Fig. 2** illustrates a calculation for a 30-year-old woman who undergoes second-trimester serum screening for Down syndrome using 3 analytes.

In the first trimester, 3 additional markers are used to screen for Down syndrome: fetal nuchal

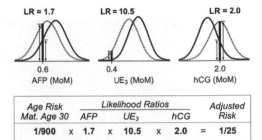

Age Risk Mat. Age 30	Likelihood Ratios AFP	UE₃	hCG	Adjusted Risk
1/900	x 1.7	x 10.5	x 2.0	= 1/25

Fig. 2. Normal distribution for 3 maternal serum analytes, AFP, UE₃, and hCG, in fetuses with Down syndrome (*dotted line*) and chromosomally normal fetuses (*solid line*) is used to illustrate calculations of LRs for each analyte. At a MSAFP level of 0.6 MoM, approximately twice as many fetuses with Down syndrome are at this level than chromosomally normal fetuses. Therefore, the LR for Down syndrome at a MSAFP level of 0.6 MoM is 1.7.

thickness measured by ultrasonography; maternal serum pregnancy-associated plasma protein A (PAPP-A) levels, which are decreased by 60% (0.43 MoM); and free β-hCG levels, which are twice as high at 1.98 MoM.[7,8] Thus, a woman who undergoes the complete integrated screen that involves first- and second-trimester markers will have 6 LRs generated for the calculation of her final AR.

FIRST-TRIMESTER ULTRASONOGRAPHIC MARKERS
Fetal Nuchal Translucency

Nicolaides and colleagues[9] described a collection of fluid at the back of the fetal neck, referred to as nuchal translucency (NT, **Fig. 3**), in the first trimester and its association with Down syndrome. The early experience with NT measurements produced a wide variation in success rates in obtaining satisfactory images and in its performance as a discriminating marker for the early diagnosis of Down syndrome. Pandya and colleagues[10] presented the first large study demonstrating the potential of first-trimester NT measurement as

Table 2
Maternal serum analyte patterns for Trisomy 21, Trisomy 18 and Neural Tube Defect.

	AFP	UE₃	hCG	Inhibin A
Trisomy 21	Increased	Increased	Decreased	Decreased
Trisomy 18	Decreased	Decreased	Decreased	—
NTD	Increased	—	—	—

The quadruple screen is completed between 15 and 20 weeks of gestation. The values are expressed in MoM to correct for the changes of these analytes with gestational age.

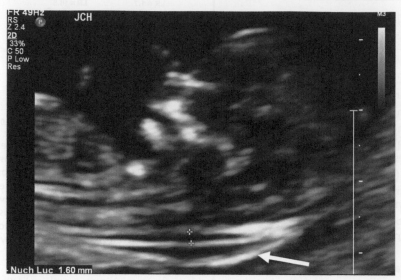

Fig. 3. The appropriate technique of measuring the NT. Arrow illustrates the amnion, and the 2 calipers are in the nuchal space measuring the NT. Both calipers have to be placed on the inside of the white line indicating the nuchal space.

a screening tool for chromosomal abnormalities. Snijders and colleagues[11] later confirmed that NT measurements could be reliably measured between 11 and 14 weeks' gestation and could be used in conjunction with maternal age to improve the detection rate for Down syndrome. The FASTER trial and the Fetal Medicine Foundation study reported the highest success rates in obtaining NT measurements on the first patient visit when the crown-rump length (CRL) was between 45 and 84 mm, which corresponds to 11 weeks 3 days and 14 weeks 2 days of gestation, respectively.[3,12] Although NT measurements can be obtained reliably and efficiently as early as 10 weeks 3 days (CRL, 36 mm), it was concluded that the benefits of obtaining the ultrasonography and NT later in the first trimester were also in confirming pregnancy viability and the identification of other anomalies such as anencephaly, abdominal wall defects, and possibly congenital heart defects.

The success of NT measurement as a screening tool whether alone or in combination with maternal serum screening hinges on the accurate procurement of images for measurement.[13,14] This is especially relevant in the evaluation of multiple gestations in which maternal serum screening is not as accurate, as in twins, or is unavailable, as in triplet or higher gestations, compared with singleton pregnancies. The detection rate for Down syndrome using NT alone is 64% to 77%, with a screen positive rate of 4.2% to 5%.[3,15] NT measurement performs better than the triple screen in the second trimester of pregnancy.

Absent Nasal Bone, Ductus Venosus, Tricuspid Regurgitation

Other first-trimester ultrasonographic findings that may be associated with Down syndrome include absent or hypoplastic nasal bone, abnormal ductus venosus flow, and tricuspid regurgitation. Cicero and colleagues[15] investigated the utility of nasal bone assessment for aneuploidy in the first trimester in a high-risk population undergoing chorionic villus sampling (CVS) and found that the nasal bone was absent in 43 of 59 fetuses (73%) with Down syndrome compared with 3 of 603 (0.5%) euploid fetuses. As expected, the calculated detection rate from this population was high at 85% at a screen positive rate of 1% (comparable to the risk of CVS). Although subsequent studies confirm the association between absent nasal bone and Down syndrome,[16–18] Malone and colleagues[19] determined that nasal bone assessment was not useful when applied in a screening program of an unselected population. The poor performance of this marker, with a sensitivity of only 7.7% and a positive predictive value of 4.5%, was in part because of the difficulty in obtaining acceptable nasal bone images. In this population of 38,189 patients, 6324 underwent nasal bone assessment, but only 76% (4801 patients) had images that were acceptable for review. There were 11 cases of Down syndrome in the nasal bone evaluation group, yet 9 of them were described as having a nasal bone and the other 2 cases were described as unable to determine. At present, the added value of the presence or absence of the nasal bone as an independent marker for a Down syndrome screening program in the general population is unclear.

Prompted by case reports of abnormal flow in the ductus venosus of chromosomally abnormal fetuses with increased NT, Matias and colleagues investigated the utility of Doppler ultrasonography assessment of the ductus venosus as a screening tool for chromosomal abnormalities in the first trimester in a high-risk population.[20,21] Absent or reverse flow was observed in 57 of 63 (90.5%) chromosomally abnormal fetuses compared with 13 of 423 (3.1%) chromosomally normal fetuses. In addition, 7 of the 13 chromosomally normal fetuses were later found to have a major cardiac defect. Subsequently, 6 studies that investigated the relationship between the ductus venosus flow and aneuploidy detected abnormal flow in 108 of 131 (82%) chromosomally abnormal fetuses, whereas only 273 of 5462 (4.9%) euploid fetuses had abnormal flow.[22] However, the studies were completed in a high-risk population and performed by experienced sonographers in maternal fetal medicine units. In the first trimester, the ductus venosus is small and less than 2 mm and Doppler waveforms can be difficult to obtain and contaminated by neighboring veins. Therefore, the application of this technique to a general-population screening program needs further investigation.

Fetal tricuspid regurgitation in the first trimester and fetal aneuploidy were found in high-risk pregnancies in which an increased NT was already detected. Huggon and colleagues[23] first studied 262 high-risk pregnancies in which 227 were referred for early echocardiography and tricuspid regurgitation was reported by pulsed Doppler in 70 (26.7%) fetuses. Of the 70 fetuses, 58 (83%) had abnormal karyotypes, whereas 68 of 192 (35%) fetuses without tricuspid regurgitation were aneuploid. Falcon and colleagues[24] found that about 70% of fetuses with Down syndrome had tricuspid regurgitation at 11 to 14 weeks' gestation and those with tricuspid regurgitation also had increased NT, elevated levels of first-trimester maternal serum β-hCG, and decreased levels of maternal serum PAPP-A. When tricuspid regurgitation detection was combined with fetal NT thickness and first-trimester maternal serum biochemical examination, the detection rate for Down syndrome was as high as 90% to 95% for a screen positive rate of 5%. Because tricuspid regurgitation determination in the first trimester is time consuming and requires expert operators, the investigators suggested a 2-stage approach to screening in the first trimester, in which, detection of tricuspid regurgitation can be reserved for the subgroup of pregnancies that have an intermediate risk for Down syndrome after completion of the first-trimester NT and maternal serum screening. In a previous multicenter study of 75,821 women who underwent only first-trimester screening, only 16% constituted the intermediate group for additional assessment of the fetal tricuspid valve.[25] More recently, in a retrospective analysis of 870 fetuses from a study group with a median maternal age of 34 years, assessments for NT thickness, nasal bone presence or absence, ductus venosus flow reversal, and tricuspid regurgitation that were completed in the early second trimester (14–18 weeks) without second-trimester maternal serum screening had a detection rate of 83.5% for Down syndrome and 100% for trisomies 18 and 13.[26]

In summary, NT measurements are routinely offered at present in first-trimester ultrasonography of the fetus. Standardization for the systematic acquisition of NT measurements and specific training with ongoing audits for quality of images have allowed the implementation of this technique by general practitioners with good detection rates. However, in studies of nasal bone, ductus venosus, and tricuspid regurgitation, the assessments were conducted by highly experienced sonographers in a selected high-risk population. Consequently, the high detection rates reported with these markers represent the best performance for each marker and put into question the practical utility of incorporating these markers into a general-population screening program.

PRENATAL SCREENING—CHOICES FOR PATIENTS

Screening is the systematic application of a test to identify asymptomatic individuals at sufficient risk for a specific disorder to benefit from further investigation or direct preventive action. The medical condition for which screening is recommended should be well defined, be of significant medical severity, and have a known incidence. Management options should be available. The screening test should be cost-effective, simple and safe, readily available, and accessible and should have a well-defined performance. In prenatal diagnostic screening programs, there should be timely transfer of test results, respect for the ethical values and decisions of patients and their family, and maximization of options for the family and fetus. Currently, there are 7 possible screening approaches in the United States for Down syndrome (**Table 3**).

Ideally, all women should be (1) offered aneuploidy and NTD screening before 20 weeks of pregnancy regardless of maternal age, (2) counseled about the nature of the conditions for which

Table 3
Approaches for screening for Down syndrome in the United States

Name	Description
Triple Screen	MSAFP, UE_3, and hCG
Quad Screen	MSAFP, UE_3, hCG, and inhibin A
Combined First-Trimester Screening	NT, maternal serum PAPP-A, and free β-hCG
Integrated Screen	NT and maternal serum PAPP-A in the first trimester, and quad screen in the second trimester; the final result is disclosed at the completion of all the tests
Serum-Only Integrated Screen	Maternal serum PAPP-A in the first trimester, and quad screen in the second trimester
Stepwise Sequential Screen	Combined first-trimester screen and quad screen with results disclosed after each test; if the first is test is negative, the patient undergoes the quad screen, with the final risk assessment incorporating the first and second results
Contingent Sequential Screen	Combined first-trimester screen with disclosure of the result. An intermediate risk is between 1:30 and 1:1500 and the patient continues to the quad screen with the final risk assessment incorporating first and second results. A negative risk is less than 1:1500 and no further screening is applied. A positive risk is greater than 1:30 and invasive testing is offered

screening is performed (NTD, Down syndrome, trisomy 18), and (3) informed about the detection rates; screen positive rates; advantages, disadvantages, and limitations of screening; and the risks and benefits of diagnostic procedures.[3] The patient's choice of screening depends on many factors and includes the personal values, perception of risk and severity of the conditions, and perception and understanding of the risk of screen positive results and the risks of invasive procedures. Counseling patients to meet these informed consent goals is intensive, time consuming, and often involves genetics professionals to provide the appropriate counseling. The ability to offer first-trimester, second-trimester, and combined screening strategies depends on the availability of certified sonographers to complete the NT measurement, the availability of CVS and/or genetic amniocentesis, and an efficient and error proof system of obtaining, tracking, and reporting results in a timely manner. Finally, the actual choice of screening test depends on the gestational age at entry to prenatal care, presence of multiple gestations, and desire for early test results versus maximal detection rate.

Candidates for second-trimester serum screening only include women who present to prenatal care after the first trimester, women who have had a first-trimester CVS but still need second-trimester screening for NTD with measurement of MSAFP only, and women with twin gestation for which the quad screen has sufficient

experience to provide reasonable detection rates. The quad screen has essentially superseded the triple screen, although rarely, in some communities, the latter is still the only second-trimester screening option.

FIRST-TRIMESTER SCREENING: COMBINED FIRST-TRIMESTER SCREENING

The screening options in the first trimester are robust. Although NT measurements alone have a high detection rate, detection rates for Down syndrome are improved substantially when NT measurements are used in combination with first-trimester maternal serum analytes PAPP-A and free β-hCG.[3,27] In the 2003 report from the First Trimester Maternal Serum Biochemistry and Fetal Nuchal Translucency Screening (BUN) study group, the overall detection rate for Down syndrome in 8514 singleton pregnancies from an unselected population was 78.7% with a 5% screen positive rate at a risk cutoff value of 1:129.[27] At a cutoff value of 1:270, which is used in second-trimester screening, the detection rate was 85.2%, but the false-positive rate was higher at 9.4%. Combined first-trimester screening detected 10 of 11 cases of trisomy 18, yielding a detection rate of 90.9%, with a false-positive rate of 2%. These detection rates are similar to those subsequently generated by the FASTER trial in which the detection rates for first-trimester combined screening were 87% at 11 weeks, 85%

at 12 weeks, and 82% at 13 weeks, with a false-positive rate of 5%.[3] The differences in detection rates between 11 and 13 weeks reflect the variation in the discriminatory power of first-trimester markers (NT and serum markers) at different gestational ages. The performance of PAPP-A is best between 8 and 11 weeks of gestation, whereas free β-hCG has the highest discriminatory value at 13 weeks.[25] In a large retrospective study, Kagan and colleagues[28] investigated different first-trimester screening strategies with the intent to maximize detection not only for aneuploidy but also for other anomalies. In a strategy for first-trimester combined screening in which ultrasonography and blood test are completed on the same day, the detection rates for Down syndrome at a screen positive rate of 5% were 94% at 11 weeks, 90% at 12 weeks, and 83% at 13 weeks. The decline in screening efficiency with increasing gestational age is caused by both fetal NT and serum PAPP-A. Therefore, the implication of these findings in designing a screening program for Down syndrome is that the best gestational age for biochemical testing and ultrasonography is 11 weeks. However, late–first-trimester ultrasonography can identify fetal abnormalities other than NT as well.[29] In an alternative strategy in which maternal blood was obtained at 10 weeks and NT measurement was performed at 12 weeks to take advantage of the larger fetus to screen for other anomalies, the detection rate for Down syndrome was 96% with a screen positive rate of 5%. Although this second 2-step first-trimester screening strategy performed better than the 1-visit strategy, the potential advantage is likely to be diminished by patient noncompliance to a second visit and by the cost of implementation. However, this study did not evaluate the detection rate of other structural abnormalities in this large cohort.

The role of NT evaluation in only dichorionic twin pregnancies is well established.[30,31] In dichorionic twins, the risk for each fetus is calculated based on the patient's age-specific risk for Down syndrome and the LR based on the deviation of the NT from the appropriate normal median for the CRL. Using this strategy, the detection rate was found to be 75% to 80%, with a screen positive rate of 5% for each fetus.[31] This screening strategy is also applied to multifetal gestations and is particularly relevant in the decision of fetal reduction for which the optimum time to be performed with the least risk to the pregnancy is 10 to 12 weeks' gestation. Patients have the option to immediately direct fetal reduction to the fetus with increased NT or, if available, proceed with CVS. Maymon and colleagues[32] compared first-trimester NT screening with second-trimester triple screening

in 60 twin and 120 singleton gestations and found a higher screen positive rate (15%) in the latter than the former (5%). In addition, the screen positive rate for the NT screen group was lower than the control group of singleton pregnancies that underwent second-trimester maternal serum screening. The higher screen positive rate in the twin pregnancies that underwent second-trimester serum screen translates into an amniocentesis rate of 15%. However, although this implies that more amniocenteses are completed, the risk of amniocentesis is less than 1:400 for loss compared with the risk of 1:100 for loss in CVS. Furthermore, because of the complexity of the procedure, CVS is not readily available in all communities.

Focus on applying the combined first-trimester screening approaches in singleton pregnancies to twin pregnancies has generated several promising findings. Spencer and Nicolaides[33] implemented first-trimester NT and maternal serum screening to 230 twin pregnancies (460 fetuses) and found an overall acceptance rate of 97.4% for screening. The detection rate for Down syndrome was 75% (3 of 4 fetuses). The risk for Down syndrome was calculated for each fetus based on the individual fetal NT and the maternal serum biochemical examination. The screen positive rate was 9% (19 of 206 pregnancies), and the uptake for invasive testing was 59% (10 of 17), with 8 patients opting for CVS and 2 for amniocentesis. More recently, Cleary-Goldman and colleagues[34] tested the utility of adding nasal bone evaluation in 2094 twin pregnancies (4188 fetuses) that were undergoing first-trimester combined screening. All sonographers who performed ultrasonography for NT and nasal bone assessment were certified in imaging. In this study, the addition of nasal bone measurement to screening increased the detection rate to 79% to 89% at a 5% screen positive rate.

In monochorionic twins, other pathologic mechanisms unique to monozygotic twinning, such as twin-twin transfusion syndrome (TTTS), and structural malformations increase the false-positive rate of NT screening. In a retrospective study of 769 monochorionic twin pregnancies that had undergone NT screening, Vandecruys and colleagues[35] found 6 fetuses with Down syndrome, 1 with trisomy 18, and 1 with triple-X. The NT measurement was in the 95th percentile or beyond in only 10.5% of chromosomally normal fetuses but in 83.3% of fetuses with Down syndrome. Increased NT was observed in both fetuses in 66.7% of these twin pregnancies. About 33% of pregnancies had an increased NT in 1 fetus. However, the average NT for CRL between the 2 fetuses in each affected pregnancy was in the 95th percentile or beyond in all 6 cases of Down syndrome. It was concluded that in monochorionic twins, effective screening for Down syndrome can be achieved by using the average of NT measured in the 2 fetuses, with a detection rate of 100% at a screen positive rate of 4.2%. It is important to point out that while discordant chromosomal abnormalities in monochorionic twins are rare, because they are, by definition, monozygotic, case reports have described discordant karyotypes in such pregnancies.[36–40] In addition, because of the increased risk for discordancy in structural malformations and TTTS, the finding of 1 twin with a normal NT should prompt the search for other causes.

For most women, the results of first-trimester screening are reassuring and in many cases, allow the disclosure of the pregnancy. At a time when the pregnancy may still be confidential, abnormal results allow for termination of pregnancy that is both safer and more private than if performed in the second trimester. In some cases, first-trimester screening identifies an unsuspected genetic syndrome for which a lengthy and complex molecular testing extends well into the second trimester.

INTEGRATED SCREENING

The FASTER trial has validated the option of universal screening for Down syndrome and trisomy 18 in all pregnant women.[3] In the integrated screen strategy, NT measurements and maternal blood are obtained during the first visit between 11 and 14 weeks of pregnancy. A second sample is obtained in the second trimester, between 15 and 20 weeks of pregnancy, after which all marker results are converted into LRs, and the AR is calculated. The integrated screen provides a detection rate of 94% to 96%, with a screen positive rate of 5%.[3] Limitations to the universal application of this screening strategy are many and include access, time of presentation to prenatal care, availability of trained operators for NT measurement, adequate counseling, compliance of returning for a second blood draw, administrative support for patient data collection, reporting, and timely follow-up of screen positive results. In communities where first-trimester NT is not available, the combined serum-only integrated screen option can be offered, which provides a detection rate of 85% to 88%. Both of these 2-step screening options have detection rates that are superior to the second-trimester quad screen alone. However, if presentation to prenatal care is after the first trimester, women should still be offered screening with the quad screen.

A Canadian Second and First Trimester Estimation of Risk (SAFER) study for Down syndrome by MacRae and colleagues[41] investigated provider and patient choices and the screening performance of the Canadian equivalent of serum-only integrated screen, integrated screen, and quad screen over a 3.5-year period in Manitoba and southeastern Ontario. In their cohort of 8571 women, screening strategies that involved some aspect of first- and second-trimester screening were chosen 4.6 times (uptake, 82% vs 18%) more often than that in quad screen. The uptake was 18% for quad screen; 46%, serum-only integrated screen; and 36%, integrated screen. The overall detection rate for the combination of screening protocols was 91%, with an overall screen positive rate of 4.5%. In 9.7% of women who selected an integrated screening strategy, second-trimester sample was not obtained. The 3 most common reasons for incomplete integrated screening were spontaneous fetal loss (2.3%), withdrawal from the study (2.1%), and unspecified reasons (1.4%). Another 1% was reassigned to a different screening strategy most commonly because of the reassignment of gestational age. The investigators noted that although the quad screen was the government-funded standard of care for all women and was the easiest option for health care providers, requiring no change in practice pattern, its uptake was still the lowest among the screening choices. Selection of the integrated screening strategies still predominated, although there were region-specific differences; for example, in regions where NT measurement was not widely available, NT measurements were reserved for women of advanced maternal age and the serum-only integrated screen protocol was used for younger women. The SAFER study demonstrates that a high detection rate with an acceptable low screen positive rate can still be achieved in a general population undergoing different screening protocols across rural and urban communities.

SEQUENTIAL AND CONTINGENT SCREENING

Two alternative screening strategies allow the disclosure of first-trimester screening results on which to base decisions regarding further testing: sequential and contingent sequential screening. Sequential screening reports the results after the first-trimester screen, and if positive, invasive testing (CVS) is offered. If results are negative, the patient continues to the second-trimester screen and is offered genetic amniocentesis if positive. Although this schema has a high detection rate, 98% from the BUN Study and 95%

from the FASTER trial, the screen positive rate is 17% and 11%, respectively.[3,27] Contingent sequential screening is a strategy that uses the first-trimester screening result to determine the need for a second-trimester screen. In this approach, women with the highest risk from the first-trimester screen are offered invasive testing by CVS, and women with the lowest risk do not continue with second-trimester testing. Women with intermediate risks continue to second-trimester testing and complete the integrated screen; if the result is positive, amniocentesis is performed. Ball and colleagues[42] evaluated the cost-effectiveness of the 7 possible screening strategies. The triple screen is not cost-effective and should be replaced universally by the quad screen as the second-trimester serum screening strategy. Only second-trimester serum screening is still cost-effective in areas where access to ultrasonography is limited or not available. Sequential and contingent screening were both cost-effective when compared with all screening strategies because there were less women continuing on to second-trimester screening because of the high detection rate of first-trimester screening.

SUMMARY

Pregnancy is now associated with many screening options for evaluation of the genetic health of the fetus. Women are presented with screening choices for Down syndrome that are complex in risk and benefit estimations, and health care providers are presented with the responsibility of providing adequate counseling, access, and the most robust screening choices for patients. Comparative analyses of the various screening options to women who are interested in prenatal diagnosis indicate that at the screen positive rate of 5%, all screening approaches have high detection rates and can be offered to patients based on availability of resources in the community and gestational age during prenatal care.

REFERENCES

1. Merkatz IR, Nitowsky HM, Macri JN, et al. An association between low maternal serum alpha-fetoprotein and chromosomal abnormalities. Am J Obstet Gynecol 1984;148:886–94.
2. Canick JA, MacRae AR. Second trimester serum markers. Semin Perinatol 2005;29:203–8.
3. Malone F, Canick JA, Ball RH, et al. First-trimester or second-trimester screening, or both, for Down's syndrome. First-and-Second Trimester Evaluation of Risk (FASTER) Research Consortium. N Engl J Med 2005;353:2001–11.
4. ACOG Committee on Practice Bulletins. ACOG Practice Bulletin No. 77: screening for fetal chromosomal abnormalities. Obstet Gynecol 2007;109:217–27.
5. Watson WJ, Chescheir NC, Seeds JW. The role of ultrasound in evaluation of patients with elevated maternal serum alpha-fetoprotein: a review. Obstet Gynecol 1991;78:123–8.
6. SOCG Technical Update. Obstetrical complications associated with abnormal maternal serum markers analytes. J Obstet Gynaecol Can 2008;30:918–32. No. 217.
7. Cuckle H. Biochemical screening for Down syndrome. Eur J Obstet Gynecol Reprod Biol 2000;92:97–101.
8. Spencer K, Wallace EM, Ritoe S. Second-trimester dimeric inhibin A in Down's syndrome screening. Prenat Diagn 1996;16:1101–10.
9. Nicolaides KH, Snijders RJ, Gosden CM, et al. Ultrasonographically detectable markers of fetal chromosomal abnormalities. Lancet 1992;340:704–7.
10. Pandya PP, Kondylios A, Hilbert L, et al. Chromosomal defects and outcome of 1015 fetuses with increased nuchal translucency. Ultrasound Obstet Gynecol 1995;5:15–9.
11. Snijders RJ, Noble P, Sebire N, et al. UK multicentre project on assessment of risk of trisomy 21 by maternal age and fetal nuchal-translucency thickness at 10-14 weeks of gestation. Fetal Medicine Foundation First Trimester Screening Group. Lancet 1998;352:343–6.
12. Avgidou k, Papageorghiou A, Bindra R, et al. Prospective first-trimester screening for trisomy 21 in 30,564 pregnancies. Am J Obstet Gynecol 2005;192:1761–7.
13. Snijders RJ, Thom EA, Zachary JM, et al. First-trimester trisomy screening nuchal translucency measurement training and quality assurance to correct and unify technique. Ultrasound Obstet Gynecol 2002;19:353–9.
14. Nicolaides KH. Nuchal translucency and other first-trimester sonographic markers of chromosomal abnormalities. Am J Obstet Gynecol 2004; 191:45–67.
15. Cicero S, Curcio P, Papageorghiou A, et al. Absence of nasal bone in fetuses with trisomy 21 at 11-14 weeks of gestation: an observational study. Lancet 2001;358:1665–7.
16. Odibo AO, Sehdev HM, Dunn L, et al. The association between fetal nasal bone hypoplasia and aneuploidy. Obstet Gynecol 2004;104:1229–33.
17. Orlandi F, Boardp CM, Campogrande M, et al. Measurement of nasal bone length at 11–14 weeks of pregnancy and its potential role in Down Syndrome risk assessment. Ultrasound Obstet Gynecol 2003;22:36–9.

18. Viora E, Masturzo B, Erranate G, et al. Ultrasound evaluations of fetal nasal bone at 11 to 14 weeks in a consecutive series of 1906 fetuses. Prenat Diagn 2003;23:784–7.

19. Malone FD, Ball RH, Nyberg DA, et al. FASTER Research Consortium. First-trimester nasal bone evaluation for aneuploidy in the general population. Obstet Gynecol 2004;104:1222–8.

20. Matias A, Gomes C, Flack N, et al. Screening for chromosomal abnormalities at 10-14 weeks: the role of ductus venosus blood flow. Ultrasound Obstet Gynecol 1998;12:380–4.

21. Matias A, Montenegro N, Areias JC, et al. Anomalous fetal venous return associated with major chromosomopathies in the late first trimester of pregnancy. Ultrasound Obstet Gynecol 1998;11:209–13.

22. Nicolaides KH, Spencer K, Avgidou K, et al. Multicenter study of first-trimester screening for trisomy 21 in 75,821 pregnancies: results and estimation of the potential impact of individual risk-oriented two-stage first-trimester screening. Ultrasound Obstet Gynecol 2005;25:221–6.

23. Huggon IC, DeFigueiredo DB, Allan LD. Tricuspid regurgitation in the diagnosis of chromosomal anomalies in the fetus at 11-14 weeks of gestation. Heart 2003;89:1071–3.

24. Falcon O, Auer M, Gerovassili A, et al. Screening for trisomy 21 by fetal tricuspid regurgitation, nuchal translucency and maternal serum free β hCG and PAPP-A at 11+0 to 13+6 weeks. Ultrasound Obstet Gynecol 2006;27:151–5.

25. Spencer K, Souter V, Tul N, et al. A screening program for trisomy 21 at 10–14 weeks using fetal nuchal translucency, maternal serum free beta-human chorionic gonadotropin and pregnancy-associated plasma protein A. Ultrasound Obstet Gynecol 1999;13:231–7.

26. Giepel A, Willruth A, Vieten J, et al. Nuchal fold thickness, nasal bone absence or hypoplasia, ductus venosus reversed flow and tricuspid valve regurgitation in screening for trisomies 21, 18 and 13 in the early second trimester. Ultrasound Obstet Gynecol 2010;35:535–9.

27. Wapner R, Thom E, Simpson JL, et al. First-trimester screening for trisomies 21 and 18. First Trimester Maternal Serum Biochemistry and Fetal Nuchal Translucency Screening (BUN) Study Group. N Engl J Med 2003;349:1405–13.

28. Kagan KO, Wright D, Baker A, et al. Screening for trisomy 21 by maternal age, fetal nuchal translucency thickness, free beta-human chorionic gonadotropin and pregnancy-associated plasma protein A. Ultrasound Obstet Gynecol 2008;31:618–24.

29. Souka AP, Pilalis A, Kavalakis Y, et al. Assessment of fetal anatomy at the 11–14 week ultrasound examination. Ultrasound Obstet Gynecol 2004;24:730–4.

30. Pandya PP, Hilbert F, Snijders RJ, et al. Nuchal translucency thickness and crown-rump length in twin pregnancies with chromosomally abnormal fetuses. J Ultrasound Med 1995;14:565–8.

31. Sebire NJ, Snijders RJ, Hughes K, et al. Screening for trisomy 21 in twin pregnancies by maternal age and fetal nuchal translucency thickness at 10-14 weeks of gestation. Br J Obstet Gynaecol 1996; 103:999–1003.

32. Maymon R, Dreazen E, Rozinsky S, et al. Comparison of nuchal translucency measurement and second-trimester triple serum screening in twin versus singleton pregnancies. Prenat Diagn 2000;20:91–5.

33. Spencer K, Nicolaides KH. Screening for trisomy 21 in twins using first trimester ultrasound and maternal serum biochemistry in a one-stop clinic: a review of three years experience. BJOG 2003; 110:276–80.

34. Cleary-Goldman J, Rebarber A, Drantz D, et al. First-trimester screening with nasal bone in twins. Am J Obstet Gynecol 2008;199:283,e1–3.

35. Vandecruys H, Failoa S, Auer M, et al. Screening for trisomy 21 in monochorionic twins by measurement of fetal nuchal translucency thickness. Ultrasound Obstet Gynecol 2005;25:551–3.

36. Machin GA. Some causes of genotypic and phenotypic discordance in monozygotic twin pairs. Am J Med Genet 1996;61:216–28.

37. Nieuwint A, Van Zalen-Sprock R, Hummel P, et al. 'Identical' twins with discordant karyotypes. Prenat Diagn 1999;19:72–6.

38. O'Donnell CP, Pertile MD, Sheffield LJ, et al. Monozygotic twins with discordant karyotypes: a case report. J Pediatr 2004;145:406–8.

39. Souka AP, Snijders RJ, Novakov A, et al. Defects and syndromes in chromosomally normal fetuses with increased nuchal translucency thickness at 10-14 weeks of gestation. Ultrasound Obstet Gynecol 1998;11:391–400.

40. Souka AP, Kraml E, Bakalis S, et al. Outcome of pregnancy in chromosomally normal fetuses with increased nuchal translucency in the first trimester. Ultrasound Obstet Gynecol 2001;18:9–17.

41. MacRae AR, Chodirker BN, Davies GA, et al. Second and first trimester estimation of risk for Down syndrome: implementation and performance in the SAFER study. Prenat Diagn 2010;30:459–66.

42. Ball RH, Caughey AB, Malone FD, et al. First- and second-trimester evaluation of risk of Down syndrome. Obstet Gynecol 2007;110:10–7.

Second-Trimester Genetic Sonogram and Soft Markers

Sarah A. Waller, MD[a],*, Theodore J. Dubinsky, MD[b],
Manjiri Dighe, MD[b]

KEYWORDS
- Genetic sonogram • Soft markers • Aneuploidy

DIAGNOSING ANOMALIES IN THE SECOND TRIMESTER ALONG WITH MINOR MARKERS AND THEIR SIGNIFICANCE

Ultrasonography was first used in 1958 by Dr Ian Donald for obstetric imaging. Over the course of the last 50 years, it has become increasingly essential in the practice of prenatal diagnosis and standard practice to recommend to patients that they undergo a screening sonogram between 18 and 22 weeks of gestation.

This recommendation evolved over the course of the last 25 years. In 1986, researchers in Finland randomly assigned 4691 women to screening ultrasonography between 16 and 20 weeks. In addition, they selected 4619 controls who underwent obstetrically indicated ultrasound procedures only. Seventy-seven percent of the women in the control group did have an ultrasonogram at some time during their pregnancy. The investigators concluded that routine second-trimester ultrasound screening was associated with an increased detection of fetal anomalies and a reduction in the perinatal mortality rate (4.6/1000 vs 9.0/1000 in controls).[1]

In 1993, the Routine Antenatal Diagnostic Imaging Ultrasound Study (RADIUS) was designed and performed. It was the first and largest randomized clinical trial to assess the effectiveness of routine ultrasound screening for women who are at low risk for poor pregnancy outcomes in the United States. The investigators randomly assigned 15,000 women to either screening ultrasonography at both 15 to 22 weeks and 31 to 35 weeks, or to ultrasonography for obstetric indications only. Forty-five percent of the control group had at least one ultrasonogram. It was concluded that routine second-trimester sonograms were associated with increased detection of fetal anomalies (34.8% vs 11%). However, the study found that there was no improvement in any perinatal outcome and no improvement in survival among anomalous fetuses. In addition, no increase in the number of terminations of pregnancy in the studied groups was observed.[2]

Finally, in 1999 Grandjean and colleagues[3] prospectively analyzed women who were routinely screened by trained sonologists between 18 and 22 weeks of gestation at 61 centers across Europe. The investigators identified 3685 anomalies, which equated to a sensitivity of routine second-trimester ultrasound screening of 56.2%. The detection rate for major anomalies was 73.7%. It was concluded that screening ultrasonography did not greatly increase the cost of prenatal care, and provided information on fetuses with anomalies prior to delivery.

Over the years many have questioned the accuracy of ultrasonography in pregnancy. The procedure greatly depends on the operator, equipment, maternal habitus, fetal gestational age, and position, and whether a standard or detailed examination is being performed. Many researchers have concluded that the prenatal detection rate for cardiac defects ranges from about 15% in low-risk populations to 80% in high-risk groups.[4–6]

[a] Division of Obstetrics and Gynecology, University of Washington, School of Medicine, 1959 NE Pacific Street, Box 356460, Seattle, WA 98195, USA
[b] Department of Radiology, University of Washington, School of Medicine, 1959 NE Pacific Street, Box 3571125, Seattle, WA 98195, USA
* Corresponding author.
E-mail address: sawaller@u.washington.edu

Ultrasound Clin 6 (2011) 11–24
doi:10.1016/j.cult.2011.01.004
1556-858X/11/$ – see front matter © 2011 Elsevier Inc. All rights reserved.

Furthermore, the optimal time to schedule patients for an anatomic survey is 20 weeks (range 16–24 weeks). This time window allows one to obtain the required views, to interpret the images, and to define normality. In 1999, a retrospective study investigating the percentage of scans that could be completed at 18, 20, and 22 weeks was completed. Schwarzler and colleagues[7] concluded that the optimal time was 20 to 23 weeks and that there was no difference in the detection rate of anomalies.

Most recently, in 2009 Thornburg and colleagues[8] completed a retrospective review of 7000 anatomy ultrasonograms that were stratified by body mass index (BMI; weight in kilograms divided by height in meters squared, ie, kg/m^2). The investigators concluded that visualization of fetal anatomy decreased with increasing BMI. This group recommended delaying anatomic survey until later than 20 weeks for women with a BMI greater than 35.

Genetic Sonogram

Ultrasonography has been proven to be a useful tool for identifying fetuses with aneuploidy. This identification is accomplished by evaluating the fetus for the presence or absence of various soft markers and major anomalies that either increase or decrease a patient's risk for an anomaly. The accepted sensitivity of second-trimester ultrasonography ranges from 13.3% to 82.4% depending on the nature of the population studied.[9] Approximately 33% of all anomalies identified are of the central nervous system, with two-thirds of those indentified having additional abnormalities. Sensitivity is dependent on various factors including the soft markers indentified, gestational age at which it is completed, maternal history, the quality of the ultrasonography performed, and the experience of those performing and reading it.[10]

Second-trimester ultrasonography has some advantages over serum screening, but most of the time it is used in conjunction with the various screening modalities, including the integrated and quadruple screens, to assess patients' risk and subsequently aid them in deciding about proceeding with diagnostic testing. Specifically, the advantages of a genetic sonogram are its ability to be used in the second trimester as well as into the third depending on the patient and situation, the ability to detect structural anomalies and the increased number of aneuploidy markers that have been identified, as well as the increased patient satisfaction by being able to see their fetus.[11]

Detection and false-positive rates vary with the type and number of markers assessed (Table 1), as well as gestational age at the time of assessment. One must remember that many normal fetuses will exhibit soft markers as well, and that identification is not a diagnosis of aneuploidy.

Structural Abnormalities

The general population has a baseline risk of 3% of having a fetus with any anomaly. The incidence of various structural abnormalities may be estimated, but one must remember that it may be an overestimation or underestimation for the specific population being considered. Many of the data gathered from birth certificate databases may have variations in definitions of certain defects as well as completeness of records. A list of selected incidences, from highest to lowest incidence, is given in Tables 2 and 3.[12]

Performance of the Ultrasonography

The guidelines followed in the United States are those set by the American Institute of Ultrasound in Medicine in 2007.[13] Within the section on fetal anatomy, the following is included: cerebellum, choroid plexus, cisterna magna, lateral cerebral ventricles, midline falx, cavum septum pellucidum, upper lip, 4-chamber view of the ear with outflow tracts if technically feasible, stomach, kidneys, urinary bladder, fetal umbilical cord insertion site, umbilical cord vessel number, intactness of the abdominal wall, cervical, thoracic, lumbar and sacral spine, and presence of upper and lower extremities. Sex of the fetus is to be documented only if medically indicated.

Soft Markers

Choroid plexus cysts
A choroid plexus cyst (CPC) is a round, cystic area found within the choroid plexus; it should be

Table 1
Isolated versus multiple sonographic markers for trisomy 21

	Trisomy 21	Normal	LR
No markers	31%	87%	0.4
1 marker	23%	11%	2
2 markers	15%	2%	10
≥3 markers	15%	0.1%	115

Abbreviation: LR, likelihood ratio.
Adapted from Breathnach FM, Fleming A, Malone FD. The second trimester genetic sonogram. Am J Med Genet Part C Semin Med Genet 2007;145C:68; with permission.

Table 2 Incidence of malformation (per 1000 live births)	
Cardiac (all)	5.6
Central nervous system (all)	4.3
Hydronephrosis	3.2
Cleft lip and/or palate	1.9
Clubbed foot/feet	1.6
Hydrocephalus	1.2
Spina bifida	1.1
Anencephaly	0.9
Abdominal wall defect	0.9
Unilateral cystic renal disease	0.6
Diaphragmatic hernia	0.5
Polycystic kidney disease	0.4
Bilateral renal agenesis	0.3

Adapted from Goldberg JD. Routine screening for fetal anomalies: expectations. Obstet Gynecol Clin North Am 2004;31:35–50; with permission.

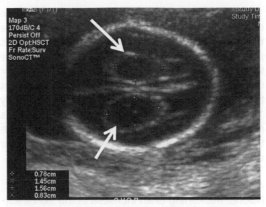

Fig. 1. Fetus with bilateral choroid plexus cysts (*arrows*).

greater than 2 mm to be considered significant (**Fig. 1**).[14] Embryologically, choroid plexus evolves from the medial wall of the lateral ventricles at around 6 weeks' gestation. Cystic spaces are formed by entanglement of villi allowing cerebrospinal fluid (CSF) to become trapped; maximum villus formation is from 13 to 18 weeks' gestation, and this is when most cysts are identified on ultrasonography. The spaces regress as the amount of stroma reduces. Usually by 28 weeks' gestation, the majority of cysts have resolved.

CPCs occur in approximately 1% to 2% of all pregnancies in isolation.[14–17] There is no ethnic prevalence and there is no strong association with trisomy 21.[15,18–21] Even though fetuses with trisomy 21 can have a CPC, this is probably a reflection of the normal distribution of CPCs in fetuses, versus an increased risk. Furthermore, there is no strong association with other aneuploidies besides trisomy 18; they have been reported in trisomy 13 and Turner syndrome. CPCs are found in approximately 40% to 60% of fetuses with trisomy 18.[18,22–24]

Ultrasonography is an excellent means of prenatally detecting trisomy 18 (67%–100% depending on gestational age). Yeo and colleagues[21] completed a retrospective case series from 1992 to 2002 in which there were 38 fetuses with trisomy 18 with a median gestational age of 20.1 (range 14.6–36.3) weeks, and all had 4 or more sonographic abnormalities. Furthermore, Picklesimer and colleagues[22] completed a retrospective review from 2000 to 2004 in which all ultrasound examinations of 36 fetuses with trisomy 18 were analyzed. It was found that between 14 and 17 weeks' gestation, 30% had no anomaly or markers visualized; however, between 18 and 24 weeks and greater than 24 weeks, all cases had abnormal ultrasonograms.[23]

Identifying an isolated CPC does not increase one's likelihood ratio significantly for aneuploidy; however, it is slightly higher than a normal anatomic survey. Walkinshaw,[25] in a meta-analysis, determined that in an unselected population a woman's risk of trisomy 18 with an isolated CPC was 1 in 189 (0.52%), and in a selected population (such as advanced maternal age) that the risk was slightly higher, at 1 in 129 (0.78%).

Table 3 Detection rates of various malformations	
Malformation	Rate (%)
Anencephaly	99.4
NTD with hydrocephalus	94.6
Hydrocephalus	93.5
Hydronephrosis	93.4
Unilateral cystic renal disease	91.7
Polycystic kidneys	91.4
Central nervous system (all)	88.3
Bilateral renal agenesis	83.7
Abdominal wall defect	81.6
NTD without hydrocephalus	66.3
Diaphragmatic hernia	58
Heart (all)	27.7
Cleft lip and/or palate	18
Clubbed foot/feet	17.2

Abbreviation: NTD, neural tube defect.
Adapted from Goldberg JD. Routine screening for fetal anomalies: expectations. Obstet Gynecol Clin North Am 2004;31:35–50; with permission.

Laterality should not be taken into account when counseling patients. There is no clear evidence that unilateral versus bilateral changes a woman's risk of aneuploidy. The literature seems to agree that prediction of trisomy 18 based on size of CPC is inappropriate, but many studies report there being larger CPCs in fetuses with trisomy 18. Because it is well known that choroid cysts resolve by approximately 28 weeks, a follow-up ultrasonogram is not recommended unless other anomalies are identified at the same time.[26–30]

Nuchal thickening

Nuchal thickening is an increase in the skin thickness at the level of the posterior fetal neck. It was first described by Landon in 1866 in fetuses with trisomy 21, and is a common marker in almost all centers in the United States for trisomy 21. The measurement should be taken between 15 and 22 weeks with an angled plane, including the cavum septum pellucidum, the cerebral peduncles, and cerebellar hemispheres (**Fig. 2**). Measurement should be obtained using transverse view through the fetal head, from the outer aspect of the occipital bone to the outer aspect of the skin edge. The upper limit of normal is 5 mm up to 20 weeks of gestational age.[31]

On average, 0.7% of normal fetuses will have nuchal skin fold measurement of 5 mm or greater. It has been associated with trisomy 21 as well with trisomy 18, triploidy, Noonan syndrome, congenital cardiac disease, and early hydrops. Its association with trisomy 21 has been shown to have a likelihood ratio of 11 to 58,[32] with a sensitivity of 7% to 75% and specificity of 98.6% to 99.5%. Prospective studies, which have used a cut-off of 5 mm or more for identification, have shown a better sensitivity with only a slight increase in false-positive rate (**Table 4**).[31,33–38] Furthermore, studies have now shown that nuchal thickness varies with gestational age and thus normograms

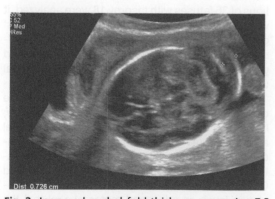

Fig. 2. Increased nuchal fold thickness measuring 7.3 mm in a fetus with known trisomy 21.

should be used to better determine significance (**Tables 5–7**).[39]

It is important to remember that factors such as dolicocephaly, breech presentation, and presence of nuchal cord are also associated with thicker nuchal fold.

Ventriculomegaly

Major or structural abnormalities of the central nervous system include holoprosencephaly, Dandy-Walker malformation, vermian agenesis, and neural tube defects. These types of abnormalities significantly increase the risk of aneuploidy. Ventriculomegaly is the term given when the measurement of the diameter of the lateral ventricular atrium is 10 mm or more (**Fig. 3**), and deserves separate consideration because it has been associated with trisomy 21 as well as other aneuploidies. Ventriculomegaly can be caused by obstruction, dysgenesis, or atrophy. One must remember that hydrocephalus is a pathologic dilation of the ventricles caused by increased pressure.[40,41]

Ventriculomegaly occurs in 1.4 to 20 per 1000 live births, with a male to female ratio of 3:1. Ninety percent of cases of ventriculomegaly are idiopathic. It is often associated with Chiari malformations, agenesis of the corpus callosum, or vein of Galen malformations, as well as those structural abnormalities previously mentioned. In 4% to 14% of cases, it is associated with aneuploidy.[40,41]

The ultrasonographic diagnosis is determined by the internal wall-to-wall measurement. On average, between 15 and 40 weeks of gestation, the mean ventricular diameter is 7 mm with 10 mm as the upper limit of normal. It is important to remember that asymmetry may occur and that unilateral ventriculomegaly is rare.

The risk associated with mild ventriculomegaly is uncertain and the majority of fetuses have no long-term sequelae,[40–47] unless associated with other structural anomalies.

Nasal bone hypoplasia/aplasia

Nasal bone hypoplasia is a soft marker for trisomy 21 in the second trimester. Studies have shown that 43% of fetuses with trisomy 21 have an absent nasal bone (**Fig. 4**) at their 15- to 22-week sonogram compared with 0.3% to 1% of normal fetuses.[24,48] Nasal bone hypoplasia is not associated with other genetic disorders. The difficulty arises because researchers and clinicians alike use different definitions for this marker. Some describe absence or presence, whereas others refer to nasal bone length as less than the 10th centile, nasal bone less than the 2.5th centile, or

Table 4
Summary of various cut-offs for abnormal nuchal fold

	≥6 mm (95% CI)	≥5 mm	≥4 mm
Sensitivity	33.3% (12%–55%)	77.8% (59%–97%)	100
Positive predictive value	75% (45%–100%)	31.8% (18%–46%)	8.2% (5%–12%)
False positive	0.1% (2/1424)	2.1%	14% (12%–16%)
Adjusted PPV	1:3	1:19	1:97

Abbreviations: CI, confidence interval; PPV, positive predictive value.
 Data from Refs.[31,33–38,49]

2 standard deviations below the mean, or even a biparietal diameter/nasal bone ratio of 11 or more.[49] It is important to remember that nasal bone size differs across ethnicities as well, which complicates interpretation and leads to greater false-positive rates. In an observational study in 2001 published in *The Lancet*, it was shown that hypoplastic nasal bones were seen in 0.5% of Caucasians and 8.8% of Afro-Caribbeans in the population examined.[50,51]

The Society for Obstetricians and Gynaecologists of Canada (SOGC) Clinical Practice Guidelines, which define hypoplasia as less than 2.5th centile, provide an overall likelihood ratio of trisomy 21 of 51. Cusick and colleagues[52] examined their population and determined that the sensitivity of an absent nasal bone as a soft marker was 55.5% with a specificity of 99.5%, giving a positive predictive value of 83.3% for trisomy 21. However, when examining hypoplastic and absent nasal bones together, they found a sensitivity of 77.7% and specificity of 99.3%. With a strong likelihood ratio, a normal nasal bone measurement may offset the marginal increase in fetal Down syndrome risk associated with other, weaker markers of aneuploidy.

Echogenic intracardiac focus
Echogenic intracardiac focus (EIF) is defined as a focus of increased echogenicity, compared with bone, in the region of the papillary muscle in either or both ventricles of the fetal heart (**Fig. 5**).[53,54] The finding of an echogenic intracardiac focus at the time of genetic sonogram has been found to correlate with mineralization within a papillary muscle.[55] An EIF is seen in 2.4% to 4.7% control fetuses in the mid-trimester.[35,36,49,56] EIFs are seen most commonly in the left ventricle.[57,58] The incidence of an EIF varies with ethnicity. In 2005, Tran and colleagues[59] concluded, in a study in which race was reported by the patient, that EIFs were found in 4.1% of all fetuses at the mid-trimester. Subdividing by race, EIFs were seen in 6.7% of African Americans, 6.9% of Asian Americans, 8.1% of

Table 5
Normogram of nuchal skin fold thickness for each gestational week in the chromosomally normal population (N = 2114)

GA (weeks)	n	Mean (mm)	95% CI of Mean	SD (mm)	10th Centile (mm)	50th Centile (mm)	90th Centile (mm)	95th Centile (mm)
16	123	2.8	2.7–2.9	0.8	2	3	4	4
17	488	3	2.9–3.1	0.9	2	3	4	5
18	705	3.3	3.2–3.4	0.9	2	3	4.1	5
19	335	3.6	3.5–3.7	0.9	2	3.2	5	5
20	155	3.7	3.5–3.9	1	2	4	5	5
21	1571	3.9	3.8–4.1	1.1	3	4	5	6
22	84	4.1	3.9–4.3	1.1	3	4	5	6
23	40	4.4	4.1–4.8	1	3	4	6	6
24	23	4.3	3.9–4.7	1	3	4	6	6

Abbreviations: CI, confidence interval; GA, gestational age; SD, standard deviation.
 Adapted from Tannirandorn Y, Manotaya S, Uerpairojkit B, et al. Cut-off criteria for second-trimester nuchal skinfold thickness for prenatal detection of Down syndrome in a Thai population. Int J Gynaecol Obstet 1999;65(2):137–41; with permission.

Table 6
Fetal pelviectasis classified according to the gestational age

15–20 weeks	$\geq$4 mm
20–30 weeks	$\geq$5 mm
>30 weeks	$\geq$7 mm

Data from Refs.[71–73]

Middle Easterners, and only 3.3% of Caucasians. However, Borgida and colleagues[60] found in their population an incidence of 5.5% in the African American population and 10.3% in the Asian population. It is widely accepted that Asians have a higher incidence of identified EIFs as compared with Caucasians, ranging from 5% to 12% in most studies.

Sonographically, detection of an EIF depends on a variety of factors, including resolution of the

sonographic equipment, technique, thoroughness of the examination, and the sonographer's experience. Fetal position is also important, because intracardiac foci are best visualized when the cardiac apex is oriented toward the transducer.[61] The SOGC recommends using an appropriate transducer frequency ($\leq$5 MHz) and appropriate gain setting, and states that an EIF can be diagnosed on the standard 4-chamber view of the fetal heart.

Identification of an EIF does increase one's risk of trisomy 21, but the exact degree varies greatly. It is well established that EIFs are seen in 18% to 30% of fetuses with Down syndrome. It is seen in isolation in only 5.4% to 9.4% of such fetuses.[35,36,56] In addition, it has been shown to be associated with fetuses with trisomy 13. Lehman and colleagues[62] reported an EIF in 30% of fetuses with trisomy 13 with an ultrasonogram before 23 weeks' gestation and 39% with

Table 7
Summary of sonographic markers of aneuploidy

Trisomy 21	Structural anomalies	Soft markers
	Cardiac abnormalities	Nuchal fold thickening
	Duodenal atresia	Ventriculomegaly
	Brachycephaly	Short humeri or femurs
	Hydrocephalus	Hypoplastic nasal bone
	Clinodactyly	Echogenic bowel
	Cystic hygroma/hydrops	Pelviectasis
		Sandal gap toe
Trisomy 18	Cardiac abnormalities	Choroid plexus cysts
	Esophageal atresia	Enlarged cisterna magna
	Strawberry-shaped head	Ventriculomegaly
	Diaphragmatic hernia	Short humeri or femurs
	Omphalocele	Hypoplastic nasal bone
	Meningomyelocele	Echogenic bowel
	Agenesis corpus callosum	Pelviectasis
	Facial clefting	Single umbilical artery
	Rocker bottom feet	
	Radial aplasia	
	Overlapping digits	
	Umbilical cord cyst	
	Cystic hygroma/hydrops	
Trisomy 13	Cardiac abnormalities	Echogenic intracardiac foci
	Diaphragmatic hernia	Enlarged cisterna magna
	Omphalocele	Ventriculomegaly
	Holoprosencephaly	Pelviectasis
	Facial clefting	Single umbilical artery
	Cyclopia	
	Agenesis corpus callosum	
	Rocker bottom feet	
	Polydactyly	
	Talipes	
	Cystic hygroma/hydrops	

Adapted from Breathnach FM, Fleming A, Malone FD. The second trimester genetic sonogram. Am J Med Genet Part C Semin Med Genet 2007;145C:62–72; with permission.

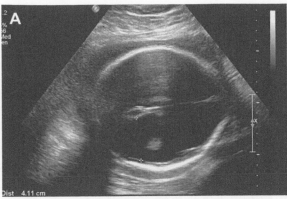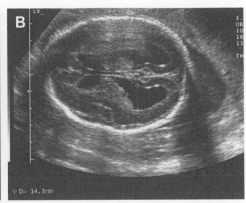

Fig. 3. Ventriculomegaly. (*A*) Severe ventriculomegaly in a fetus with acqueductal stenosis with ventricles measuring 4.1 cm in size. Note almost complete lack of cortical tissue. (*B*) Mild ventriculomegaly in a fetus with suspected trisomy 13 with ventricles measuring 14 mm in size.

ultrasonograms between 12 and 20 weeks of gestation. All of these fetuses had additional anomalies detected, although they were subtle in 2 cases.

An isolated EIF provides a likelihood ratio of 1 to 2 based on consensus from multiple studies. By contrast, some have suggested that either a right-sided or multiple EIFs are further risk

factors and that amniocentesis should be offered to patients. Bromley and colleagues[57,58] concluded that right-sided and bilateral EIF combined had approximately a twofold greater risk for aneuploidy than left-sided foci. At the authors' institution, if an EIF is seen it is reported, but as an isolated finding no further ultrasonography, including echocardiography, is required.

Echogenic bowel

Echogenic bowel, first described in 1992 by Dicke and Crane, is defined as a homogeneous, hyperechogenic area in the lower abdomen corresponding to the fetal bowel, which does not shadow and usually resolves within a few weeks with no long-term sequelae to the fetus (**Fig. 6**).[63] Bowel is considered hyperechoic if it appears identical to

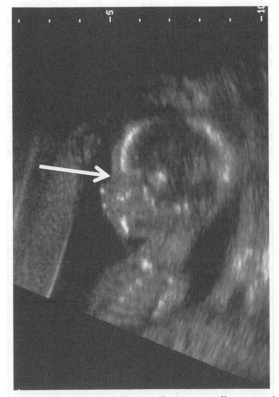

Fig. 4. Absent nasal bone. Chromosomally normal fetus with absent nasal bone (*arrow*).

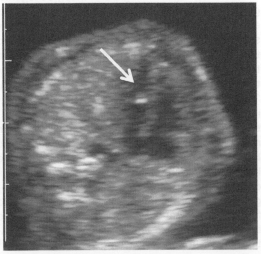

Fig. 5. Echogenic intracardiac focus (EIF). Echogenic focus seen within the left ventricle consistent with an EIF (*arrow*).

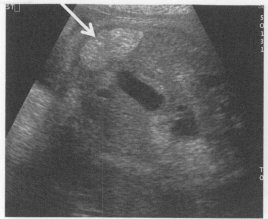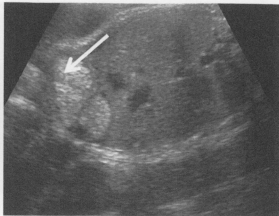

Fig. 6. Echogenic bowel with increased echogenecity compared to liver and bone (*arrows*).

the adjacent bone and brighter than the liver. Some have hypothesized that echogenic bowel is caused by decreased swallowing, hypoperistalsis, bowel obstruction, hypercellular meconium, swallowing of intra-amniotic blood, or bowel hypotonia with desiccation of meconium. In normal fetuses, bowel peristalsis begins at 15 weeks' gestation and meconium is present in the small bowel at 16 to 18 weeks' gestation. It is a common finding in many third-trimester ultrasonograms, with grade 2 or 3 echogenic bowel being seen in 1.2% (range 0.2%–1.8%) of fetuses scanned in the mid-trimester.

As echogenic bowel was being identified more frequently, the need for a classification system developed. In 1993, Nyberg and colleagues[64] compared the echogenicity of bowel to that of the liver. These investigators referred to grade 0 as isoechoic (normal); grade 1 mildly echogenic; grade 2 moderately echogenic; and grade 3 markedly echogenic and nearly as echogenic as bony structures. In using this system, they concluded that "no variation in interpretation involved more than one grade level and little interobserver variation was encountered in differentiating grades 2 or 3 bowel echogenicity from grades 0 or 1, suggesting that experienced sonologists can reliably identify hyperechoic bowel and distinguish it from normal bowel echogenicity." Whenever echogenic bowel is suspected, the gain setting should be lowered and harmonics turned off to enable this comparison and to ensure that bowel hyperechogenicity is real. If grade 1 is suspected, then no further investigations are required. Echogenic bowel is detectable as early as 14 weeks' gestation, but the mean time at diagnosis is 18 weeks.[49]

Echogenic bowel is described in many cases of trisomy 21 (4.7%), cystic fibrosis (3.5%), and in utero infections (3.2%), as well as other chromosomal (2.6%) and structural anomalies (**Box 1**). In 2001 Nyberg and Souter[61] found that 17.2% of fetuses with Down syndrome have grade 2 or 3 echogenic bowel and that 3.2% of fetuses with trisomy 21 have this as an isolated finding. In 2003, Simon-Bouy and colleagues[65] found that 2.5% of fetuses with grade 2 to 3 echogenic bowel were subsequently diagnosed with Down syndrome. In 1992, Dicke and Crane[63] found that 13.3% of fetuses with persistent echogenic bowel were diagnosed postnatally with cystic fibrosis. However, in 2000 Strocker and colleagues[66] identified 91 fetuses with echogenic bowel, none of which were born with cystic fibrosis by clinical examination. This study was limited in that genetic analysis and long-term follow-up was unavailable.

Fetuses of mothers who acquire viral illnesses during pregnancy compose another large proportion of cases of isolated echogenic bowel. In 2000, Strocker and colleagues[66] reviewed 131 cases of

---

Box 1
Causes of echogenic bowel

Bleeding

Aneuploidy

Congenital infection

Meconium ileus (cystic fibrosis)

Growth restriction

Bowel obstruction/atresia

α-Thalassemia (rare)

Data from Nyberg DA, Souter VL. Use of genetic sonography for adjusting the risk for fetal Down syndrome [review]. Semin Perinatol 2003;27(2):130–44.

isolated echogenic bowel and concluded there was a 10% infectious etiology, which in turn was attributed to multiple causes. Through a series of confirmatory clinical tests they identified varicella, rubella, parvovirus, herpes simplex virus, cytomegalovirus, and gram-negative sepsis as causes of echogenic bowel. This review was followed by a study by Simon-Bouy and colleagues[65] in 2003, who found that 2.8% fetuses with grade 2 to 3 echogenic bowel had an in utero fetal infection, but could only isolate cytomegalovirus and parvovirus as sources. Several additional studies have reaffirmed that cytomegalovirus and parvovirus are the most common infectious agents.

The final group of fetuses who are seen to have echogenic bowel are those with other chromosomal and structural anomalies. This group is a diverse one, which includes trisomy 18,[63] triploidy,[64] and Turner syndrome.[49] Structurally, echogenic bowel is seen in fetuses with gastrointestinal abnormalities such as imperforate anuses, cardiac anomalies,[64,66] and α-thalassemia minor.[67,68]

Fetuses diagnosed with echogenic bowel as an isolated marker should be followed throughout the pregnancy, as they are at risk for growth restriction and fetal demise. Strocker and colleagues[66] found that 6.9% of fetuses with echogenicity similar to or greater than bone and who had a normal karyotype developed fetal growth restriction. Ghose and colleagues[69] found that 10% of fetuses with echogenicity similar to or greater than surrounding fetal bone developed growth restriction, and 4 subsequently died perinatally. Furthermore, Al-Kouatly and colleagues[70] identified 9 of 156 (5.8%) fetuses with unexplained echogenic bowel (normal karyotype, no structural abnormalities, no cystic fibrosis mutations, no evidence of infection) who had a fetal demise. In this cohort, elevated maternal serum α-fetoprotein was the strongest predictor of demise and growth restriction, and oligohydramnios was commonly seen.

Pelviectasis
Mild pelviectasis is a common finding, often incidental, with no significant long-term complications or sequelae. Dilation of the fetal renal pelvis is a common finding during second-trimester anatomic surveys, with an incidence of 0.3% to 4.5% (average around 1%).[71] Mild pelviectasis is diagnosed when the renal pelvis measures 4 mm or more and less than 10 mm in the anteroposterior dimensions in axial scans of the abdomen at the second-trimester sonogram (**Fig. 7**). This condition varies slightly as gestation increases (see **Table 1**).[71–73] The incidence of pelviectasis during normal pregnancy is between 4.5% and

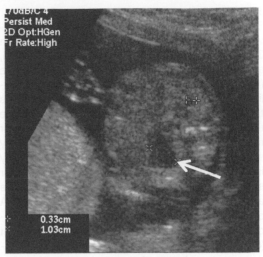

Fig. 7. Pelviectasis. 20 week old fetus with unilateral pelviectasis measuring 10 mm (*arrow*).

7%. Male fetuses exhibit a significantly increased frequency of renal pelvis dilatation as compared with females (3:1). Fetal pelviectasis can be unilateral or bilateral, but is more frequently reported as bilateral and is more common on the left side. Fetuses with significant pelviectasis (hydronephrosis if ≥10 mm) are at risk for having renal structural abnormalities, which would require a postnatal evaluation. Although the incidence of pelviectasis and calyceal dilatation is higher in boys, the outcome of the two sexes is similar. Mothers with fetal pelviectasis in their first pregnancy have a relative risk of 6 to 1 for a recurrence in subsequent pregnancies.[71]

When pelviectasis is identified, clinicians must recognize that 4 to 10 mm is clinically relevant. However, in 80% of those cases between 4 and 7 mm, there is complete resolution; 7 to 10 mm are of intermediate range, with most resolving prenatally; and 30% to 40% of those greater than 10 mm require a postnatal evaluation and, occasionally, intervention by pediatric nephrology. The majority of cases resolve spontaneously within the first year of life, requiring only monitoring and prophylactic antibiotics. Reflux is the most common morbidity that is long-standing. Clinically a follow-up sonogram is recommended between 28 and 32 weeks if pelviectasis is identified.[71–78]

As an isolated finding, pelviectasis should not increase one's baseline or serum screening risk; however, if identified, a careful survey for other soft markers should be completed, because there is no clear consensus on the incidence of Down syndrome (14%–35%) when fetal pelviectasis is isolated. However, it is important to recognize that 25% of fetuses with trisomy 21 have pelviectasis.[75,77]

Single umbilical artery

Single umbilical artery (SUA) is defined as a 2-vessel cord as compared with the more common 3-vessel cord with 2 arteries and a single vein, and occurs in 0.25% to 1% of pregnancies (**Fig. 8**). SUA is associated with other fetal anomalies including cardiac and renal defects. It is thought to occur as thrombotic atrophy of one umbilical artery, primary agenesis of an artery, or the persistence of the allantoic artery in the early stages of embryonic life. It is believed that atrophy is the most frequent mechanism. The latter scenario, when both arteries close and the vitelline artery persists, corresponds to about 1.4% of SUA cases, and is associated with sirenomelia. Hypoplasia of one of the arteries is less frequent (0.03%) and is associated with fetal growth restriction, maternal diabetes, polyhydramnios, and congenital cardiomyopathy. To date, it remains unclear why fetuses with isolated SUA have poorer perinatal outcomes than normal fetuses. It has been demonstrated that these cords have a lower number of spirals and less Wharton jelly, which might make them less resistant in situations of stress, such as birth or compression of the umbilical cord.[79–88]

SUA can be diagnosed as early as 13 weeks' gestation. When the diagnosis of SUA is made, a detailed fetal anatomy survey is indicated. If fetal anomalies are detected, further diagnostic testing such as amniocentesis may be warranted. Some investigators recommended fetal echocardiogram if SUA is an isolated finding[79,80]; however, others ascribe to no further evaluation.[81] In cases of isolated SUA there is no indication for fetal karyotyping, because there is no evidence of increased risk of aneuploidy. Associations have been made with chromosome abnormalities, specifically trisomies 13 and 18, as well as triploidy, but no clear link has been identified. However, it is well known that perinatal morbidity is increased in fetuses with a SUA, specifically growth restriction, and close obstetric observation and testing as indicated is warranted in such cases.

Shortened long bones

Shortened humeri and femurs have been associated with trisomy 21. A shortened long bone is defined as a measurement obtained that is less than the 2.5th centile for the specific gestational age. In a recent meta-analysis, shortened femurs provided a likelihood ratio of 2.7.[56] In the same study, shortened humeri have a likelihood ratio of 7.5 for Down syndrome. It is important to remember that shortened long bones are also markers of nonchromosomal abnormalities such as skeletal dysplasias and growth restriction.[11,32,36]

Other Markers

Other potential clinical markers have been suggested and studied in wide array; however, they have not been adopted in routine clinical practice.[53,54] These markers include:

- Fifth-finger clinodactyly: a hypoplastic or absent mid-phalanx of the fifth digit
- Brachycephaly: the abnormal skull shape that results from shortening of the frontal occipital brain length primarily owing to a smaller frontal lobe in fetuses with trisomy 21
- Increased iliac angle: wider lateral flare of the iliac bone
- Small fetal ear length: fetal ear position is difficult to determine sonographically but normal ranges have been established.

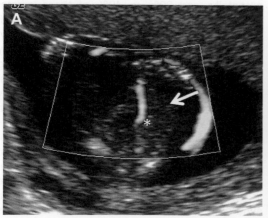
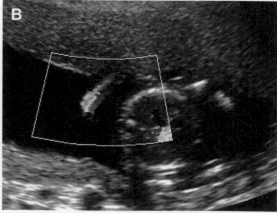

Fig. 8. Single umbilical artery. Fetus with single umbilical artery (*arrow*) seen around the bladder (*asterisk*) on a cross-section through the fetal pelvis (*A*) and a longitudinal section through the cord (*B*) showing a single artery (*blue*) and vein (*red*) in the cord.

Adverse Effects of Genetic Ultrasound

There have been multiple long-term studies in the United States and internationally that have not shown any increased risk of adverse outcomes to the fetus. The harm that comes from routine ultrasound screening is the false-positive rate associated with it, as well as the identification of soft markers that may or may not increase one's risk of an anomaly or aneuploidy; this can affect a woman's decision whether to continue a pregnancy or pursue termination. It is very important to instruct all patients that ultrasonography is not 100% accurate and that it cannot detect all cases of aneuploidy.

SUMMARY

Techniques in ultrasonography have improved dramatically over the last several years. Ultrasonography provides patients with an excellent means of screening for anomalies, and the use of soft markers has individualized each patient's decision to pursue diagnostic testing. Consensus across disciplines, including radiology and obstetrics, is that a combined modality of maternal age, serum screening, and ultrasonography provides patients the best risk assessment. One must keep in mind the limitations of technology during the search for further noninvasive diagnostic tools in this field. A normal ultrasonogram reduces the risk of trisomy 21 by 60% to 70% (likelihood ratio of 0.3–0.4) but does not completely negate it.[10]

REFERENCES

1. Saari-Kemppainen A, Karjalainen O, Ylöstalo P, et al. Ultrasound screening and perinatal mortality: controlled trial of systematic one-stage screening in pregnancy. The Helsinki Ultrasound Trial. Lancet 1990;336(8712):387–91.
2. Crane JP, LeFevre ML, Winborn RC, et al. A randomized trial of prenatal ultrasonographic screening: impact on the detection, management, and outcome of anomalous fetuses. The RADIUS Study Group. Am J Obstet Gynecol 1994;171(2):392–9.
3. Grandjean H, Larroque D, Levi S. The performance of routine ultrasonographic screening of pregnancies in the Eurofetus Study. Am J Obstet Gynecol 1999;181(2):446–54.
4. Benacerraf BR, Gelman R, Frigoletto FD Jr. Sonographic identification of second-trimester fetuses with Down syndrome. N Engl J Med 1987;317(22):1371–6.
5. Crawford DC, Chita SK, Allan LD. Prenatal detection of congenital heart disease: factors affecting obstetric management and survival. Am J Obstet Gynecol 1988;159(2):352–6.
6. Ott WJ, Arias F, Sheldon G, et al. Comprehensive ultrasound examination in a private perinatal practice [review]. Am J Perinatol 1995;12(6):385–91.
7. Schwarzler P, Senat MV, Holden D, et al. Feasibility of the second-trimester fetal ultrasound examination in an unselected population at 18, 20 or 22 weeks of pregnancy a randomized trial. Ultrasound Obstet Gynecol 1999;14:92–7.
8. Thornburg LL, Miles K, Ho M, et al. Fetal anatomic evaluation in the overweight and obese gravida. Ultrasound Obstet Gynecol 2009;33(6):670–5.
9. Levi S. Ultrasound in prenatal diagnosis: polemics around routine ultrasound screening for second trimester fetal malformations. Prenat Diagn 2002;22(4):285–95.
10. Nyberg DA, Souter VL. Use of genetic sonography for adjusting the risk for fetal Down syndrome [review]. Semin Perinatol 2003;27(2):130–44.
11. Nyberg DA. Second trimester genetic sonogram—how does it fit in? 2009. Available at: http://www.miniseminaires.com/wp-content/uploads/2009/06/6-chromosal-defects.pdf. Accessed September 15, 2010.
12. Goldberg JD. Routine screening for fetal anomalies: expectations. Obstet Gynecol Clin North Am 2004;31:35–50.
13. Guidelines for obstetric ultrasound. American Institute of Ultrasound in Medicine; 2007. Available at: http://www.aium.org/publications/guidelines/obstetric.pdf. Accessed September 1, 2010.
14. Woodward P, Kennedy A, Sohaey R, et al. Diagnostic imaging obstetrics. 1st edition. Amirsys, Manitoba, Canada: 2005.
15. Bromley B, Lieberman R, Benacerraf BR, et al. Choroid plexus cysts: not associated with Down syndrome. Ultrasound Obstet Gynecol 1996;8:232–5.
16. Chitty LS, Chudleigh P, Wright E, et al. The significance of choroid plexus cysts in an unselected population: results of a multicenter study. Ultrasound Obstet Gynecol 1998;12:391–7.
17. Verdin SM, Whitlow BJ, Lazanakis M, et al. Ultrasonographic markers for chromosomal abnormalities in women with negative nuchal translucency and second trimester maternal serum biochemistry. Ultrasound Obstet Gynecol 2000;16(5):402–6.
18. Devore GR. Second trimester ultrasonography may identify 77–97% of fetuses with trisomy 18. J Ultrasound Med 2000;19:565–76.
19. Bronsteen R, Lee W, Vettraino IM, et al. Second trimester sonography and trisomy 18. J Ultrasound Med 2004;23:241–5.
20. Gupta JK, Khan KS, Thornton JG, et al. Management of fetal choroid plexus cysts. Br J Obstet Gynaecol 1997;104:881–6.
21. Yeo L, Guzman ER, Day-Salvatore D, et al. Prenatal detection of fetal Trisomy 18 through abnormal

sonographic features. J Ultrasound Med 2003;22: 581–90.

22. Picklesimer A, Moise KJ Jr, Wolfe HM, et al. The impact of gestational age on the sonographic detection of aneuploidy. Am J Obstet Gynecol 2005;193:1243–7.

23. Papp C, Szigeti Z, Tóth-Pál E, et al. Ultrasonographic findings of fetal aneuploidies in the second trimester—our experiences. Fetal Diagn Ther 2008; 23:105–13.

24. Bethune M. Literature review and suggested protocol for managing ultrasound soft markers for Down syndrome: thickened nuchal fold, echogenic bowel, shortened femur, shortened humerus, pyelectasis and absent or hypoplastic nasal bone [review]. Australas Radiol 2007;51(3):218–25.

25. Walkinshaw SA. Fetal choroid plexus cysts: are we there yet? Prenat Diagn 2000;20:657–62.

26. Coco C, Jeanty P. Karyotyping of fetuses with isolated choroid plexus cysts is not justified in an unselected population. J Ultrasound Med 2004;23:899–906.

27. Yoder PR, Sabbagha RE, Gross SJ, et al. The second trimester fetus with isolated choroid plexus cysts: a meta-analysis of risk of Trisomies 18 and 21. Obstet Gynecol 1999;93(5):869–72.

28. Beke A, Barakonyi E, Belics Z, et al. Risk of chromosome abnormalities in the presence of bilateral or unilateral choroid plexus cysts. Fetal Diagn Ther 2008;23:185–91.

29. Demasio K, Canterino J, Ananth C, et al. Isolated choroid plexus cyst in low-risk women less than 35 years old. Am J Obstet Gynecol 2002;187:1246–9.

30. Ghidini A, Strobelt N, Locatelli A, et al. Isolated fetal CPC: role of ultrasonography in establishment of risk of trisomy 18. Am J Obstet Gynecol 2000;182(4): 972–7.

31. Benacerraf B. The significance of the nuchal fold in the second trimester fetus. Prenat Diagn 2002;22: 798–801.

32. Nyberg DA, Resta RG, Luthy DA, et al. Prenatal sonographic findings in Down syndrome. Review of 94 cases. Obstet Gynecol 1990;76:370–7.

33. Vintzileos AM, Campbell WA, Guzman ER, et al. Second-trimester ultrasound markers for detection of trisomy 21: which markers are best? Obstet Gynecol 1997;89:941–4.

34. Grandjean H, Sarramon MF. Sonographic measurement of nuchal skinfold thickness for detection of Down syndrome in the second-trimester fetus: a multicenter prospective study. The AFDPHE Study Group. Association Française pour le Dépistage et la Prévention des Handicaps de l'Enfant. Obstet Gynecol 1995;85(1):103–6.

35. Nyberg DA, Luthy DA, Resta RG, et al. Age-adjusted ultrasound risk assessment for fetal Down syndrome during the second trimester: description of the method and analysis of 142 cases. Ultrasound Obstet Gynecol 1998;12:8–14.

36. Nyberg DA, Souter VL, El-Bastawissi A, et al. Isolated sonographic markers for detection of fetal Down syndrome in the second trimester of pregnancy. J Ultrasound Med 2001;20:1053–63.

37. Borrell A, Farré MT, Echevarría M, et al. Nuchal thickness evolution in trisomy 18 fetuses. Ultrasound Obstet Gynecol 2000;16(2):146–8.

38. Gray DL, Crane JP. Optimal nuchal skin-fold thresholds based on gestational age for prenatal detection of Down syndrome. Am J Obstet Gynecol 1994; 171(5):1282–6.

39. Tannirandorn Y, Manotaya S, Uerpairojkit B, et al. Cut-off criteria for second-trimester nuchal skinfold thickness for prenatal detection of Down syndrome in a Thai population. Int J Gynaecol Obstet 1999; 65(2):137–41.

40. Pilu G, Falco P, Gabrielli S, et al. The clinical significance of fetal isolated cerebral borderline ventriculomegaly: report of 31 cases and review of the literature. Ultrasound Obstet Gynecol 1999;14:320–6.

41. Achiron R, Schimmel M, Achiron A, et al. Fetal mild idiopathic lateral ventriculomegaly: is there a correlation with fetal trisomy? Ultrasound Obstet Gynecol 1993;3:89–92.

42. Cardoza JD, Goldstein RB, Filly RA. Exclusion of fetal ventriculomegaly with a single measurement: the width of the lateral ventricular atrium. Radiology 1988;169:711–4.

43. Filly RA, Cardoza JD, Goldstein RB, et al. Detection of fetal central nervous system anomalies: a practical level of effort for a routine sonogram. Radiology 1989;172:403–8.

44. Nicolaides KH, Berry S, Snijders RJ, et al. Fetal lateral cerebral ventriculomegaly: associated malformations and chromosomal defects. Fetal Diagn Ther 1990;5(1):5–14.

45. Signorelli M, Tiberti A, Valseriati D, et al. Width of the fetal lateral ventricular atrium between 10 and 12 mm: a simple variation of the norm? Ultrasound Obstet Gynecol 2004;23:14–8.

46. Lipitz S, Yagel S, Malinger G, et al. Outcome of fetuses with isolated borderline unilateral ventriculomegaly diagnosed at mid-gestation. Ultrasound Obstet Gynecol 1998;12(1):23–6.

47. Senat MV, Bernard JP, Schwarzler P, et al. Prenatal diagnosis and follow-up of 14 cases of unilateral ventriculomegaly. Ultrasound Obstet Gynecol 1999;14(5):327–32.

48. Bromley B, Lieberman E, Shipp TD, et al. Fetal nose bone length: a marker for Down syndrome in the second trimester. J Ultrasound Med 2002;21(12): 1387–94. Erratum appears in J Ultrasound Med 2003;22(2):162.

49. Bromley B, Lieberman E, Shipp TD, et al. The genetic sonogram a method of risk assessment for down syndrome in the second trimester. J Ultrasound Med 2002;21:1087–96.

50. Cicero S, Sacchini C, Rembouskos G, et al. Sonographic markers of fetal aneuploidy—a review [review]. Placenta 2003;24(Suppl B):S88–98.
51. Cicero S, Curcio P, Papageorghiou A, et al. Absence of nasal bone in fetuses with trisomy 21 at 11–14 weeks of gestation: an observational study. Lancet 2001;358(9294):1665–7.
52. Cusick W, Shevell T, Duchan LS, et al. Likelihood ratios for fetal trisomy 21 based on nasal bone length in the second trimester: how best to define hypoplasia? Ultrasound Obstet Gynecol 2007;30(3):271–4.
53. Van den Hof MC, Wilson RD. Fetal soft markers in ultrasound. Diagnostic Imaging Committee, Society of Obstetricians and Gynaecologists of Canada; Genetics Committee, Society of Obstetricians and Gynaecologists of Canada. J Obstet Gynaecol Can 2005;27(6):592–636.
54. Van den Hof MC, Deminaczuk NN. Content of a complete obstetrical ultrasound report. J Soc Obstet Gynaecol Can 2001;23(5):427–8.
55. Brown DL, Roberts DJ, Miller WA. Left ventricular echogenic focus in the fetal heart: pathologic correlation. J Ultrasound Med 1994;13(8):613–6.
56. Smith-Bindman R, Hosmer W, Feldstein VA, et al. Second-trimester ultrasound to detect fetuses with Down syndrome: a meta-analysis. JAMA 2001;285(8):1044–55.
57. Bromley B, Lieberman E, Laboda L, et al. Echogenic intracardiac focus: a sonographic sign for fetal Down syndrome. Obstet Gynecol 1995;86:998–1001.
58. Bromley B, Lieberman E, Shipp TD, et al. Significance of an echogenic intracardiac focus in fetuses at high and low risk for aneuploidy. J Ultrasound Med 1998;17(2):127–31.
59. Tran SH, Caughey AB, Norton ME. Ethnic variation in the prevalence of echogenic intracardiac foci and the association with Down syndrome. Ultrasound Obstet Gynecol 2005;26(2):158–61.
60. Borgida AF, Maffeo C, Gianferarri EA, et al. Frequency of echogenic intracardiac focus by race/ethnicity in euploid fetuses. J Matern Fetal Neonatal Med 2005;18(1):65–6.
61. Nyberg DA, Souter VL. Sonographic markers of fetal aneuploidy. Clin Perinatol 2000;27(4):761–89.
62. Lehman CD, Nyberg DA, Winter TC 3rd, et al. Trisomy 13 syndrome: prenatal US findings in a review of 33 cases. Radiology 1995;194(1):217–22.
63. Dicke JM, Crane JP. Sonographically detected hyperechoic fetal bowel: significance and implications for pregnancy management. Obstet Gynecol 1992;80(5):778–82.
64. Nyberg DA, Dubinsky T, Resta RG, et al. Echogenic fetal bowel during the second trimester: clinical importance. Radiology 1993;188(2):527–31.
65. Simon-Bouy B, Satre V, Ferec C, et al. Hyperechogenic fetal bowel: a large French collaborative study of 682 cases. Am J Med Genet A 2003;121(3):209–13.
66. Strocker AM, Snijders RJ, Carlson DE, et al. Fetal echogenic bowel: parameters to be considered in differential diagnosis. Ultrasound Obstet Gynecol 2000;16(6):519–23.
67. Lam YH, Tang MH, Lee CP, et al. Echogenic bowel in fetuses with homozygous alpha-thalassemia-1 in the first and second trimesters. Ultrasound Obstet Gynecol 1999;14:180–2.
68. Langer B. Fetal pyelectasis. Ultrasound Obstet Gynecol 2000;16:1–5.
69. Ghose I, Mason GC, Martinez D, et al. Hyperechogenic fetal bowel: a prospective analysis of sixty consecutive cases. BJOG 2000;107(3):426–9.
70. Al-Kouatly HB, Chasen ST, Karam AK, et al. Factors associated with fetal demise in fetal echogenic bowel. Am J Obstet Gynecol 2001;185(5):1039–43.
71. Chudleigh T. Mild pyelectasis. Prenat Diagn 2001;101:936–41.
72. Benacerraf B, et al. Fetal pyelectasis: a possible association with Down syndrome. Obstet Gynecol 1990;76:58.
73. Wickstrom E, Thangavelu M, Parilla BV, et al. A prospective study of the association between isolated fetal pyelectasis and chromosomal abnormality. Obstet Gynecol 1996;88:125.
74. Adra A, Mejides AA, Dennaoui MS, et al. Fetal pyelectasis: is it always "physiologic"? Am J Obstet Gynecol 1995;6:1263–6.
75. Bornstein E, Barnhard Y, Donnenfeld AE, et al. The risk of a major trisomy in fetuses with pyelectasis: the impact of an abnormal maternal serum screen or additional sonographic markers. Am J Obstet Gynecol 2007;196(5):263–9.
76. Broadley P, McHugo J, Morgan I, et al. The 4 year outcome following the demonstration of bilateral renal pelvic dilation on pre-natal renal ultrasound. Br J Radiol 1999;72:265–70.
77. Coco C, Jeanty P. Isolated fetal pyelectasis and chromosomal abnormalities. Am J Obstet Gynecol 2005;193:290–7.
78. Ouzounian J, Castro MA, Fresquez M, et al. Prognostic significance of antenatally detected fetal pyelectasis. Ultrasound Obstet Gynecol 1996;7:424–8.
79. Lubusky M, Dhaifalah I, Prochazka M, et al. Single umbilical artery and its siding in the second trimester of pregnancy: relation to chromosomal defects. Prenat Diagn 2007;27:327–31.
80. Cristina MP, Ana G, Inés T, et al. Perinatal results following the prenatal diagnosis of single umbilical artery. Acta Obstet Gynecol Scand 2005;84(11):1068–74.
81. Bombrys A, Neiger R, Hawkins S, et al. Pregnancy outcome in isolated single umbilical artery. Am J Perinatol 2008;25:239–42.

82. Budorick NE, Kelly TF, Dunn JA, et al. The single umbilical artery in a high risk patient population: what should be offered? J Ultrasound Med 2001; 20(6):619–27.

83. Martinez-Frias M, Bermejo E, Rodríguez-Pinilla E, et al. Does single umbilical artery (SUA) predict any type of congenital defect? Clinical-epidemiological analysis of a large consecutive series of malformed infants. Am J Med Genet A 2008;146:15–25.

84. Granese R, Coco C, Jeanty P, et al. The value of single umbilical artery in the prediction of fetal aneuploidy. Ultrasound Q 2007;23(2):117–21.

85. Wiegand S, McKenna DS, Croom C, et al. Serial sonographic growth assessment in pregnancies complicated by an isolated single umbilical artery. Am J Perinatol 2008;25:149–52.

86. American College of Obstetricians and Gynecologists. Prenatal diagnosis of fetal chromosomal abnormalities. In: Clinical management guidelines for obstetrician-gynecologists. Washington, DC: American College of Obstetricians and Gynecologists; 2001. p. 4–12. Practice Bulletin 27.

87. Gabbe S, Niebyl J, Simpson J, et al. Obstetrics: normal and problem pregnancies. 5th edition. Philadelphia (PA): Churchill Livingstone; 2007. Chapter 12.

88. Gomez KJ, Copel JA. Ultrasound screening for fetal structural anomalies. Curr Opin Obstet Gynecol 1993;5(2):204–10.

Three-Dimensional Ultrasound of Fetal Orofacial Anomalies

A. Luana Stanescu, MD[a],*, Manjiri Dighe, MD[b],
Corinne L. Fligner, MD[c], Theodore J. Dubinsky, MD[b]

KEYWORDS

- Fetal • Orofacial malformations • Ultrasound
- Cleft lip/palate

A complete radiologic evaluation of the fetal face would include not just nose and lips but also the maxilla, mandible, tongue, eyes, ears, bridge of the nose, skull sutures, and shape of the forehead. Common orofacial anomalies such as cleft lip, with or without cleft palate, are seen in the United States in 6800 newborns annually, and at an incidence of 10 per 10,000 live births. Cleft palate alone occurs in approximately 6 newborns per 10,000 live births.[1] Orofacial anomalies may also suggest the presence of other accompanying malformations, warranting a careful general evaluation of the fetal anatomy. Shaw and colleagues[2] reported that 71% of patients with cleft palate and 60% of patients with cleft lip and palate had additional associated anomalies. The common teaching that the face predicts the brain is applicable to the radiologic evaluation of many intracranial anomalies, especially significant brain malformations such as holoprosencephaly, making the careful imaging of the fetal face an important part of the prenatal ultrasound examination.

Prenatal diagnosis should be targeted toward maximizing the information obtained from various modalities to detect additional structural and chromosomal anomalies in order to develop a plan for the management of the pregnancy and postnatal care of the infant. Likewise, the early detection of fetal anomalies may allow psychological and emotional preparation of the parents to alleviate postnatal anxiety related to special care appropriate to the orofacial anomaly.

This article provides an overview of the orofacial anomalies detectable by ultrasound, illustrating their appearance on imaging and associated findings.

ULTRASOUND TECHNIQUE

Ultrasound technology allows identification of major facial anomalies as early as 12 weeks.[3] However, a second-trimester ultrasound examination provides a better rate of detection and characterization of these anomalies. In our institution, images of the face are routinely acquired in coronal and sagittal planes during the second-trimester ultrasound scan. A midline sagittal scan (profile view) is useful for evaluation of the size of the mandible (allowing identification of micrognathia), nose, nasal bridge, and forehead (**Fig. 1**A). The coronal plane is used to image the lower face, particularly the nose and lips (see **Fig. 1**B). This image is acquired in a plane tangential to the anterior aspect of the lower face and should include the tip of the nose, nostrils, and upper and lower lips. Nonvisualization of the lower lip and chin on the coronal images is highly suspicious for micrognathia. Additional axial scans can be used to evaluate the upper lip/anterior palate, the oral cavity, and the orbits, allowing detection of hypotelorism, hypertelorism, anophthalmia, and other orbital and eye anomalies.[4]

Three-dimensional (3D) ultrasound provides tridimensional images of the fetal face (**Fig. 2**), and is particularly useful in the evaluation of

[a] Department of Radiology, Seattle Children's Hospital, Seattle, WA, USA
[b] Department of Radiology, University of Washington Medical Center, Box 357115, Seattle, WA 98195, USA
[c] Department of Pathology, University of Washington Medical Center, Seattle, WA, USA
* Corresponding author.
E-mail address: stanescu@u.washington.edu

Ultrasound Clin 6 (2011) 25–38
doi:10.1016/j.cult.2011.01.005

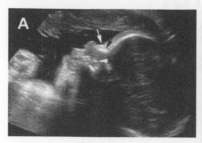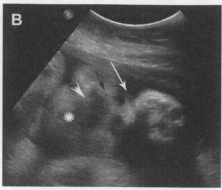

Fig. 1. Ultrasound imaging planes. (*A*) Normal profile. Transabdominal ultrasound image of the fetal profile acquired in the midline sagittal plane shows nasal bone (*black arrow*) oriented obliquely along the frontocaudal direction at approximately 45 degrees, in continuity with the frontal bone. The skin line can also appear as an echogenic line, but is more superficial and not in continuity with the frontal bone (*white arrow*). Presence and length of the nasal bone can be evaluated on this view. Upper lip imaged in this midline plane should be linear with no abnormal contour. Secondary palate is defined by a thick hyper echoic line extending from the alveolar level posteriorly (*white arrowhead*). Tongue is seen in the oral cavity. Normal frontal forehead is straight or slightly angled posteriorly. (*B*) Normal nose/lips. Transabdominal ultrasound image is acquired in a coronal plane tangential to the anterior aspect of the face and should include the tip of the nose and nostrils (*white arrow*), upper lip (*black arrow*), and lower lip (*white arrowhead*). Chin can also be seen in this view (*). A continuous echogenic upper lip excludes a cleft lip.

clefts.[5] Two techniques have been described in the literature. The reverse face technique, described by Campbell and colleagues,[6,7] uses a slow 3D sweep of the fetal profile with harmonics for high resolution and better interface definition. The acquired volume is then rotated 180 degrees to a coronal view and the plane is scrolled from back to front, allowing visualization of the secondary palate without shadowing from the maxilla. A limitation of this technique is the difficulty in evaluating the soft palate, likely caused by vertical orientation that cannot be properly evaluated in a coronal view (**Fig. 3**A). The flipped face technique, described by Platt and colleagues,[8] performs the volume sweep either in sagittal plane, from lateral to lateral sides of the face, or in axial plane from chin to nose, also with slow sweep speed and harmonics. The rendered image is then rotated to an axial plane and scrolled in sequential planes from the chin to the orbits, providing an effective method of evaluation of fetal lips, alveolar ridges, and hard and soft palates (see **Fig. 3**B). Limitations of this technique are related to adequate volume acquisition as well as shadowing from the hard palate, which also obscures visualization of the soft palate. Both techniques are reported to provide additional high value in identifying cleft palate in patients with cleft lip visualized on two-dimensional (2D) screening. More recent studies have described the usefulness of 3D techniques in the evaluation of nasal bones, metopic sutures, orbits, and ears.[5,9–13] Benoit and Chaoui[9] used 3D ultrasound to evaluate nasal bones in fetuses with Down syndrome, whereas Chaoui and colleagues[10] used 3D reconstructions with maximum transparent mode to evaluate metopic suture synostosis detected by 2D ultrasound, describing both the patterns of abnormal development and the associated defects. Chang and colleagues[12] used 3 ear parameters (height, length, and area) measured by 3D ultrasound to develop charts for ear growth related to gestational age. They suggested that these charts could be useful in increasing the rate of detection of aneuploidy when used in conjunction with other parameters.

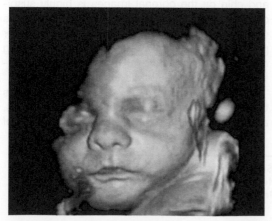

Fig. 2. Normal 3D of the face at 30 weeks, with normal eyes, nose, and lips.

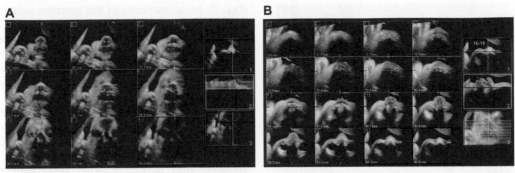

Fig. 3. 3D ultrasound techniques for evaluating the fetal face. (*A*) Reversed face technique: the acquired volume can be evaluated by scrolling through contiguous coronal slices. (*B*) Flipped face technique: the rendered image is scrolled in sequential axial planes from chin (*first rows*) to the orbits (*last rows*).

For ease of description, **Table 1** provides a classification of the major orofacial anomalies that are detectable by ultrasound and are reviewed in this article.

UPPER FACE
Orbit Anomalies

Anophthalmia and microphthalmia represent a spectrum of ocular and orbital abnormalities characterized by small size of the eyes and orbits, with anophthalmia being the most severe form of the disorder. Measurements of the orbits and ocular globes, and comparison with normograms, should be performed in all cases suggestive of eye anomalies.[14] Anophthalmia is a rare condition (0.3–0.6/10,000 births) defined by absence of optic tissue in the orbit because of failed formation of the optic vesicle. It may be isolated or associated with central nervous system anomalies, chromosomal anomalies (trisomy 13), and/or mental retardation.[15] When it presents as an isolated finding, it may represent the expression of a single-gene disorder such as Fraser syndrome (cryptophthalmos-syndactyly), Goldenhar syndrome, or hemifacial microsomia.[16] Toxoplasmosis, rubella, cytomegalovirus and herpes (TORCH) screening is indicated in all cases because of the association with cytomegalovirus and rubella infection.[14,17] Sonographic diagnosis is challenging; detailed evaluation of orbital and ocular structures is indicated when flat or concave eyelids are observed, suggesting absent ocular globes (**Fig. 4**).

Microphthalmia consists of small ocular globes (**Fig. 5**); this diagnosis can be confirmed by measurement of an orbital diameter smaller then the fifth percentile for gestational age according to the Jeanty eye growth charts, using at least 3 measurements performed in the axial and coronal planes.[18–20] Incidences reported by different investigators vary between 1 in 2400 and 1 in

---

Table 1
Orofacial anomalies detected by ultrasound

	Upper Face			Mid Face		Lower Face
Orbits and Ears	Cranium	Nose	Midfacial Hypoplasia	Lips/Palate/Tongue		Jaw/Oral Cavity
Anophthalmia/ microphthalmia	Frontal bossing	Absent nasal bones	—	Clefts		Micrognathia
Proptosis	Craniosynostosis	Hypoplastic nasal bones	—	Macroglossia Microglossia Glossoptosis		Retrognathia
Hypotelorism/ cyclopia	—	Nasolacrimal duct cysts	—	—		Tumors and masses
Hypertelorism	—	Proboscis	—	—		—
Small ears Low-set ears Dysplastic ears	—	—	—	—		—

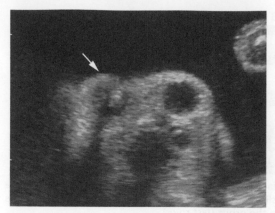

Fig. 4. Anophthalmia. Axial image at the level of the orbits shows unilateral absent ocular globe consistent with anophthalmia in a 28 weeks fetus (*arrow*).

8300 pregnancies.[18,21] Microphthalmia can be an isolated finding, a component of single-gene syndromes such as Fraser syndrome or Meckel Gruber syndrome, or it may be associated with chromosomal anomalies such as trisomy 13.[14] Exposure to radiation between 4 and 11 weeks of gestation,[22] as well as TORCH infection, have all been suggested as possible causes for of microphtalmos.[14]

Proptosis is defined as forward displacement of the eyes, assessed subjectively (**Fig. 6**). This condition may be caused by shallow orbits as a consequence of premature fusion of sutures in a skeletal dysplasia, such as Crouzon[23,24] or Apert syndromes.[25,26] Prominent ocular globes in normal bony orbits may be a sign of fetal thyrotoxicosis in maternal Graves disease, seen in association with other fetal signs of hyperthyroidism such as tachycardia and congestive heart failure.[27]

Hypotelorism represents a decreased distance between the eyes below the fifth percentile

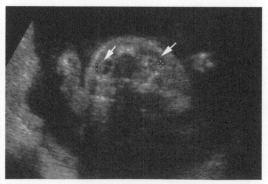

Fig. 5. Microphthalmia: axial plane at the level of the orbits shows bilateral small ocular globes in a fetus with trisomy 13 (*arrows*).

(**Fig. 7**). Measurements of the biorbital and interorbital distances can be obtained from the transverse view of the orbits and compared with normal values. According to Jeanty and colleagues,[19] the axial image for measurement should be perfectly symmetric, with both eyes equal, and the maximum diameter should be used for the measurements. Hypotelorism may be caused by restrained lateral migration of the orbits caused by metopic synostosis in craniosynostosis syndromes, and is also frequently associated with abnormal brain development in holoprosencephaly spectrum.[28] Holoprosencephaly is associated with variable degrees of hypotelorism from mild to the most severe form, which is cyclopia. Hypotelorism has been described in association with chromosomal anomalies such as trisomy 13 and 21, and may also represent a normal variant in otherwise normal individuals.[29] Maternal use of ethanol and retinoic acid–containing medications and maternal diabetes have also been linked to hypotelorism.

Cyclopia and synophthalmia are extreme forms of hypotelorism representing variable degrees of fused single median bony orbit, containing either a single eye or 2 adjacent partially fused eyes, respectively.[30] These entities are encountered in 10% to 20% of fetuses with alobar holoprosencephaly[31] as part of the spectrum of median plane malformations of the face and brain.[32] Prenatal diagnosis of alobar holoprosencephaly should trigger a search for craniofacial dysmorphism, with absence of butterfly sign of the choroid plexus on first trimester scan being an early indicator for holoprosencephaly.[33] Associated findings may include absent nasal bone, flat profile, and a proboscis (**Fig. 8**). 3D sonography may play an important role in confirming the initial 2D sonographic diagnosis; recent studies have described the value of 3D ultrasound in visualization of the fused orbit and associated findings as early as 13 weeks of gestation.[34,35] There is a high association of these entities with chromosomal anomalies, with trisomy 13 being the most common, followed by trisomy 18 and triploidy.[34,35]

Hypertelorism is an abnormally increased distance between the eyes above the 95th percentile, caused by lateral displacement of the medial orbital wall. This condition can be seen as an isolated finding (benign), in frontonasal dysplasia (isolated or syndromic), in association with encephalocele, and in oblique facial clefting. Tan and Mulliken[36] reviewed a series of 90 patients with hypertelorism and found that the most common cause was frontonasal dysplasia, followed by craniofrontonasal dysplasia. Frontonasal dysplasia

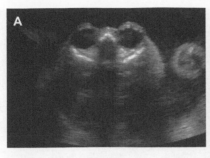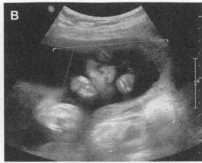

Fig. 6. Proptosis. Prominent, bulging ocular globes in a fetus with thanatophoric dysplasia on axial (A) and coronal (B) 2D ultrasound imaging.

consists of hypertelorism, as well as a broad nasal root, midline facial cleft, cleft nasal alae, hypoplastic nasal tip, and anterior cranium bifidum, with most cases being sporadic, although autosomal dominance as well as X-linked inheritance have been described.[37] Craniofrontonasal dysplasia is an X-linked malformation caused by mutations in EFNB1 gene associating coronal synostosis to the frontofacial malformations.[38]

Ears

Recent advances in 3D ultrasound account for better assessment of the fetal ear size and position (**Fig. 9**), with normograms based on several ear parameters and gestational age being established by Chang and colleagues.[12] Several studies have described a high association between small-sized ears and trisomies,[16,39,40] whereas low-set and/or malformed ears are seen in Treacher Collins syndrome,[41,42] Fraser syndrome,[43] as well as in CHARGE (Coloboma of the eye, heart defects, atresia of the choanae, retardation of growth and/or development, genital and/or urinary abnormalities, and ear abnormalities and deafness) and VACTERL (vertebrae, anus,

cardiovascular tree, trachea, esophagus, renal system, and limb buds) associations.[5]

Cranium

The fetal forehead is normally straight or slightly angled posteriorly, as opposed to frontal bossing in which there is prominence of the forehead (**Fig. 10**). This condition can be associated with achondroplasia, craniosynostosis syndromes, Meckel Gruber, and osteogenesis imperfecta caused by deficient ossification, as well as in some intracranial anomalies such as hemimegalencephaly caused by increased hydrocephalus.[29] Usually the fetal forehead is evaluated by subjective assessment on 2D ultrasound; however, objective measurements have been developed by 3D ultrasound.[44,45] Sivan and colleagues[45] generated normograms for forehead length, height, and area and calculated a forehead index based on 3D ultrasound measurements performed on a series of 130 singleton pregnancies between 16 and 38 weeks of gestation.

Craniosynostosis detection is usually triggered by an abnormal head shape on 2D ultrasound and has significantly progressed with the advent of 3D imaging.[5,16] Fetal features encountered in

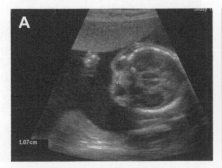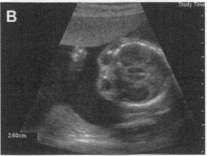

Fig. 7. Hypotelorism. (A, B) Axial plane through fetal orbits shows the orbits too close together, with the interorbital and biorbital distances measuring less than fifth percentile, corresponding to 17 weeks fetal age in a 20-week fetus with holoprosencephaly.

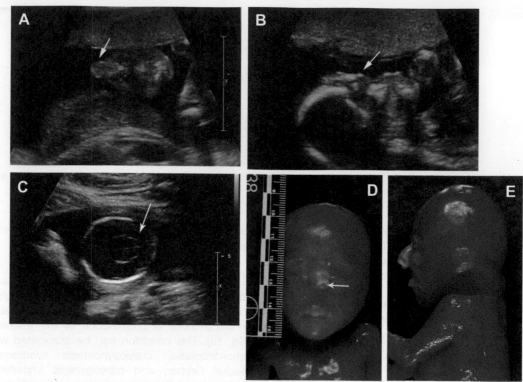

Fig. 8. Proboscis. Absence of a normal nose with presence of a rudimentary, tubular, noselike midline structure originating from the lower frontal aspect of the head, consistent with proboscis (*arrow*), visualized in coronal (*A*) and sagittal (*B*) planes in a fetus with trisomy 13 and alobar holoprosencephaly. (*C*) Axial image through the head shows a monoventricle and fused thalami (*arrow*) suggesting alobar holoprosencephaly. (*D, E*) Autopsy images showing the proboscis with absent philtrum and single nostril (*arrow*) suggesting ethmocephaly.

fibroblast growth factor receptor (FGFR)–related craniosynostosis syndromes such as Apert, Crouzon, and Pfeiffer are similar and mainly represented by midfacial hypoplasia, acrocephaly, hypertelorism, and frontal bossing.[16]

Nasal Abnormalities

Absent or short nasal bones are a common feature in trisomy 21. According to recent studies, approximately 65% of fetuses with trisomy 21 examined by ultrasound between 11 and 24 weeks showed this feature (Fig. 11).[46,47] Kagan and colleagues[47] determined that absent nasal bone can also be present in trisomy 18 (53%) and trisomy 13 (45%) and can be evaluated as part of the first trimester screening. The technique

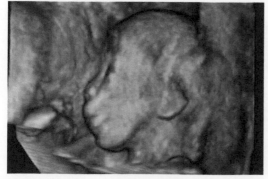

Fig. 9. Fetal ear: 3D reformat shows small, dysplastic ear in a child with Down syndrome and absent nasal bones.

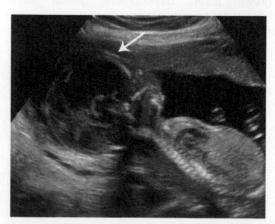

Fig. 10. Fetal forehead bossing. Prominent forehead (*arrow*) in a fetus diagnosed with osteogenesis imperfecta type II.

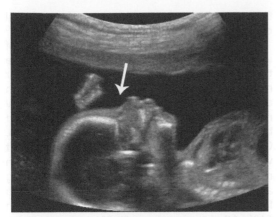

Fig. 11. Absent nasal bones. Sagittal plane image shows absent nasal bone ossification (*arrow*) in the expected location of the nasal bones in a trisomy 21 fetus.

described by Kagan and colleagues[47] is imaging the nasal bone in the midsagittal plane of the fetal head on a magnified image, with nasal bones considered to be present if more echogenic than the skin line. Improved 3D techniques are also used in evaluating nasal bones.[5,9] For example, Benoit and Chaoui[9] reported better visualization of the nasal bones with 3D ultrasound, which allows the assessment of both nasal bones, with the new observation that nasal bone hypoplasia or aplasia can be unilateral in fetuses with Down syndrome.

Nasolacrimal duct cysts (dacryocystoceles) are small, thin-walled, hypoechoic structures located anteromedially to the orbit that may be unilateral or bilateral on 2D ultrasound (**Fig. 12**). They are caused by obstruction of the lacrimal duct at both ends caused by nonpermeability of the valve system, and are usually an isolated, benign finding.[48] Differential diagnosis includes nasal glioma, frontonasal encephalocele, hemangioma,

and dermoid cysts. 3D ultrasound is a useful tool for evaluating a dacryocystocele, providing information regarding the possible intranasal extension and possibly avoiding additional investigations in the neonatal period.[49–51]

MID AND LOWER FACE
Mouth and Lip Anomalies

Clefts are the most common craniofacial malformations and are among the most common congenital abnormalities (1 in 1000 births). According to Nyberg and colleagues,[16,52] they can be classified as cleft lip unilateral, bilateral, midline cleft lip and palate, and amniotic band/slash-type defects (oblique facial clefting) (**Table 2**).

Cleft lip and palate represent approximately 50% of cases, with isolated cleft lip seen in only 20% and cleft palate in about 30%.[16] The primary palate usually fuses by 8 weeks and the secondary palate by 12 weeks of gestation.[16] However, head position and the small size of the fetal face relative to the transducer make imaging of the fetal face challenging before 15 weeks of gestation.

Isolated cleft lips (**Fig. 13**) are diagnosed by visualizing a defect in the soft tissue of the upper lip with intact alveolar ridge.[53] However, diagnosis of a cleft lip triggers a detailed evaluation of the palate in axial or coronal plane as well as with 3D reconstructions. Cleft lips are less frequently associated with syndromes or genetic aberrations than cleft palate only.

It is thought in most cases that cleft lip and palate are causally distinct from cleft palate only, with unilateral cleft lip and palate being most common and less severe than bilateral cleft lip and palate. A recent epidemiology study confirms earlier data stating that cleft lip and palate, as well as cleft lip, are more prevalent in boys, whereas cleft palate is more frequent in girls.[54]

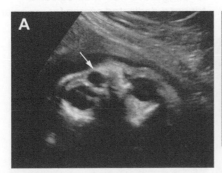
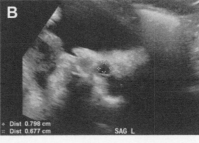

Fig. 12. Nasolacrimal duct cyst. (*A*) Axial ultrasound image at the level of the orbits shows a small, thin-walled, hypoechoic structure anteromedial to the left orbit (*arrow*). (*B*) Sagittal ultrasound image acquired in a plane medial to the left orbit shows the same thin-walled, hypoechoic structure anterior to the orbit.

Table 2
Orofacial clefts classification

Type 1	Cleft lip
Type 2	Unilateral cleft lip and palate
Type 3	Bilateral cleft lip and palate
Type 4	Midline cleft lip and palate
Type 5	Amniotic band/slash-type defects

Modified after Nyberg DA, Sickler GK, Hegge FN, et al. Fetal cleft lip with and without cleft palate: US classification and correlation with outcome. Radiology 1995; 195(3):677–84.

Unilateral cleft lip and palate can be visualized as a defect in the upper lip and alveolus on the nose/lips, axial and coronal views, and 3D.

Bilateral cleft lip and palate (**Fig. 14**A) can be categorized, depending on presence or absence of premaxillary protrusion, into 2 subgroups. The premaxillary segment protrusion (see **Fig. 14**B) is encountered in most cases and appears as a paranasal echogenic mass that may be confused with other facial masses such as anterior cephaloceles, hemangiomas, teratomas, or proboscis.[52,55] In the subgroup without protrusion, a hypoplastic midface with a depressed nose is visualized, and only the presence of a ridge of intact skin and lip in the midline can differentiate it from midline cleft lip and palate.

Midline cleft lip and palate usually carries a poor outcome because of a high association with chromosomal anomalies[3] and malformations.[16,52] The most common chromosomal abnormality associated with this type of cleft is trisomy 13.[3]

Isolated cleft palate is particularly difficult to diagnose prenatally because of the tongue as well as because of acoustic shadow from the facial bones. Indirect signs of cleft lip and palate are a small stomach and polyhydramnios caused by fetal difficulty with swallowing.[56,57] Increased tongue excursion in the absence of a cleft lip may indicate a cleft palate. Color Doppler ultrasound may be used to visualize the abnormal flow of amniotic fluid from the mouth into the nasal cavity, showing the presence of a palatal cleft.[56–58]

In a study by Nyberg,[16] more than 30% of infants born with a cleft lip and palate, and more than 50% of those with cleft palate, had other malformations. Most common malformations in association with clefts are found in the central nervous system and the skeletal system, followed by the urogenital and cardiovascular systems. Chromosomal anomalies associated with cleft vary from 0% in cleft lip to more than 52% in median cleft lip and palate according to Nyberg and colleagues.[52,55] Berge and colleagues[3] also found associated chromosomal anomalies in 51% of their case series, with 0% for isolated cleft lip, hence the cytogenetic evaluation can be valuable for cases with cleft lip and palate.

A different approach to orofacial cleft epidemiology was described by Tolarova and Cervenka,[59] who found that isolated clefts occur in 63.7% of cases, with the highest proportion in cleft lips (86%). Most nonisolated clefts (18.6%) were found to be part of a complex of multiple congenital anomalies of unknown cause.

Chromosomal aberrations were found in 8.8% of the patients with clefts, the most common being trisomy 13, whereas sequences were found in 4% of the patients, with Robin sequence representing most, followed by holoprosencephaly.

Tongue

Tongue size and motion can be assessed in both coronal and sagittal planes. Although fetal tongue normograms correlated with gestational age have been established,[60,61] the ultrasound assessment remains mainly subjective and defines the normal-sized fetal tongue as posteriorly positioned to the gums on a profile view for most of the ultrasound examination duration, with brief intermittent episodes of protrusion.[62] Persistent tongue protrusion, especially if associated with polyhydramnios, is suggestive for macroglossia[4,63] and should trigger a dedicated search for associated findings,

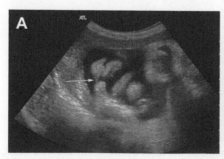
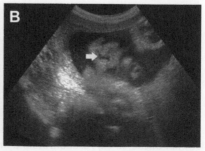

Fig. 13. Unilateral cleft lip. (*A, B*) Coronal ultrasound images tangential to nose and lips (nose/lips view) show a soft tissue defect of the upper lip with intact alveolar ridge (*arrow*).

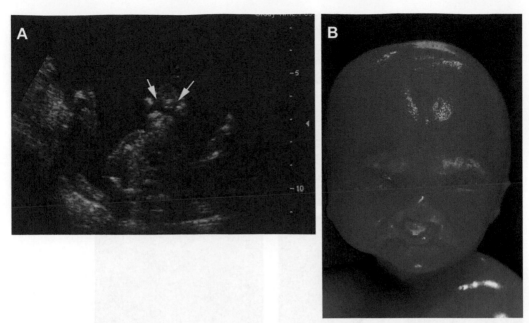

Fig. 14. Bilateral cleft lip and palate. (*A*) Coronal plane ultrasound in a 22-week fetus with trisomy 13 shows bilateral hypoechoic defects (*arrows*) in the upper lip cleft lip. Sagittal image revealed premaxillary protrusion. (*B*) A 22-week fetus with bilateral cleft lip and palate and premaxillary protrusion.

such as omphalocele, macrosomia, and enlarged kidneys, to diagnose Beckwith-Wiedemann syndrome or goiter associated with congenital hypothyroidism.[63] Macroglossia can also be encountered in trisomy 21, inborn metabolism storage disorders (like Hunter or Hurler), or can be caused by infiltrating tongue masses such as lymphangioma, hemangioma,[62,64] or, rarely, teratomas.[63,65]

Microglossia has been described in rare chromosomal anomalies such as trisomy 1.[16,60] Posterior displacement of the tongue never reaching the anterior alveolar ridge (glossoptosis) represents a feature encountered in Pierre Robin sequence and likely caused by the small-sized oral cavity and micrognathia.[16,60,66]

Mandible Anomalies

Fetal mandible abnormalities are common, with retrognathia being defined by a receding chin, whereas micrognathia is a small mandible. The importance of ultrasound detection of these defects is to provide information to the family and care providers regarding the potential of an increased risk for upper airway obstruction caused by abnormal tongue position. Micrognathia (**Fig. 15**) usually develops secondary to abnormalities of the first branchial arch by deficiency or insufficient migration of the neural crest cells in the fourth week of gestation, resulting in a small

mandible. This condition is a common feature in Robin sequence (airway obstruction, micrognathia, and glossoptosis) and Treacher Collins syndrome (downward slant of the eyes, micrognathia, hypoplastic zygomatic arches, and macrostomia),[4,16,42,67] and can be associated with trisomy 18 and, less frequently, with trisomy 21. Diagnosis is usually subjective on prenatal ultrasound: presence of a receding or small chin with a prominent upper lip on the profile view, as well as inability to see the chin on a nose/lips view, are suspicious findings (see **Fig. 15**C). However, multiple studies attempt to provide an objective measurement for mandible anomalies. Rotten and colleagues[68] described 2 parameters: the inferofacial angle is used for diagnosing retrognathia, with a mean value of 65.5 degrees and a standard deviation of 8.1 for normal values, whereas the mandible/maxilla width ratio is constant between 18 and 28 gestational weeks, with a mean normal value of 1.017 and values less 0.785 defining micrognathia. Borenstein and colleagues[69,70] used the mandibulomaxillary facial angle to identify micrognathia in fetuses with trisomy 18 as early as 11 weeks of gestation, whereas Palit and colleagues[70] introduced a frontonasal angle as an objective measurement for retrognathia. The usefulness of these measurements in 2D ultrasound may be limited by sonographer expertise, fetal position, and excessive shadowing from overlying bones, but developments in 3D

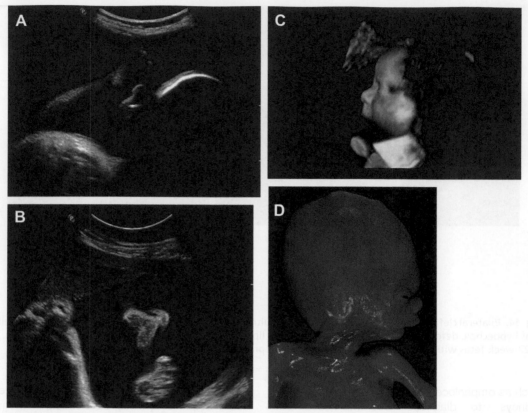

Fig. 15. Micrognathia. Profile view visualized by 2D (*A*) and 3D (*B*) ultrasound shows severe micrognathia in a 29-week fetus with Pierre Robin sequence. Nonvisualization of the chin on the nose/lips view (*C*) is also suggestive for micrognathia. (*D*) Another 25-week fetus with profound micrognathia, prominent glabella, and depressed nose bridge (from autopsy).

techniques can overcome some of these factors by allowing reformats in the appropriate plane. Ultrasound detection of fetal micrognathia is extremely important because of the high association with posterior displacement of the tongue with airway obstruction that may require intubation at delivery.

OROFACIAL TUMORS AND MASSES

Face and neck are the second most common location for fetal tumors after heart. Neither malignancy, aneuploidy, nor associated malformations are usually associated with face and neck tumors. Common orofacial tumors are oropharyngeal teratoma, oral cysts, and lymphangioma.

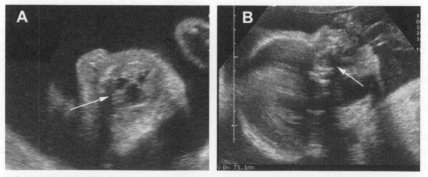

Fig. 16. Epignathus. (*A*) Nose/lips view showing a complex heterogeneous cystic and solid mass protruding through fetal mouth (*arrow*), and (*B*) ultrasound profile view showing the complex oral mass extending intracranially (*arrow*) as well as in the lower neck.

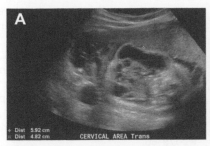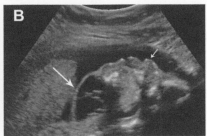

Fig. 17. Lymphangioma. (*A*) Axial image through the cervical region of a 23-week fetus shows a large, anterior, multiseptated, predominantly cystic lesion. (*B*) Sagittal image in a different fetus shows a predominantly cystic lesion (*long arrow*), partially invading the mouth floor and extending down in the cervical region. Short arrow indicates nasal tip.

Epignathus (**Fig. 16**) is a rare teratoma arising from the oral cavity and pharynx, in the region of the basisphenoid (Rathke pouch)[4,16] or from the mandible.[71] Incidence is low, ranging from 1 in 35,000 to 1 in 200,000 live births according to Smith and colleagues.[72] By definition, teratomas include at least 1 tissue type from each of the embryonic layers, so ultrasound detects a complex mass, predominantly solid. Intracranial extension is possible, so further examination with magnetic resonance is usually warranted.[71] The most commonly associated anomaly is cleft palate, believed to be caused by mechanical disruption preventing closure of the palatal shelves.[4,16] This anomaly is often associated with polyhydramnios caused by obstructed swallowing, with a poor prognosis in large tumors even if the mass is benign.[4,71] Differential diagnosis would include macroglossia, cysts (salivary), lymphangioma, and neurofibroma.[16] Antenatal diagnosis by ultrasound imaging is essential for perioperative care and management: cesarean section and further perioperative care and management, which may include an ex utero intrapartum treatment (EXIT) procedure[73] and management by a neonatal airway specialist during delivery.

Congenital cystic lesions of the oral cavity are rare. Ranula represents a mucous extravasation cyst developed following disruption of salivary glands and resultant extravasation of mucous in contiguous connective tissues,[74] whereas retention cysts result from proximal expansion of a blocked duct from the submaxillary and submandibulary glands. Heterotopic gastrointestinal cysts in the oral cavity have also been described.[75] Prenatal ultrasound detection of congenital oral cyst has been reported for only 2 cases.[76]

Lymphangiomas are congenital malformations of lymphatic vessels filled with a clear protein-rich fluid containing few lymph cells, usually diagnosed in infancy and early childhood. Oral lymphangiomas may occur at various sites, most frequently on the anterior two-thirds of the tongue, which often results in macroglossia. These lymphangiomas can also be present in the palate, buccal mucosa, gingiva, and lip.[4,16] Ultrasound appearance is of a hypoechoic, usually multilocular mass, with no flow signal on Doppler (**Fig. 17**). Depending on mass location and extension, EXIT procedure may be needed for delivery.

SUMMARY

Orofacial anomalies are common and have a high association with other fetal abnormalities. Hence, early diagnosis is important, and detailed imaging of the fetal face is an important part of ultrasound examination when evaluating the fetus at risk. Improved 3D techniques allow a better visualization of the face, as well as for deeper structures such as the hard palate, improving the rate of detection for cleft palate. Early diagnosis provides clinicians with appropriate information for further management that includes psychological preparation and education of the parents, as well as planned neonatal care.

REFERENCES

1. Canfield MA, Honein MA, Yuskiv N, et al. National estimates and race/ethnic-specific variation of selected birth defects in the United States, 1999–2001. Birth Defects Res A Clin Mol Teratol 2006; 76(11):747–56.
2. Shaw GM, Carmichael SL, Yang W, et al. Congenital malformations in births with orofacial clefts among 3.6 million California births, 1983–1997. Am J Med Genet A 2004;125(3):250–6.
3. Berge SJ, Plath H, Van de Vondel PT, et al. Fetal cleft lip and palate: sonographic diagnosis, chromosomal abnormalities, associated anomalies and postnatal outcome in 70 fetuses. Ultrasound Obstet Gynecol 2001;18(5):422–31.

4. Peter CW. Ultrasonography in obstetrics and gyne-cology. 5th edition. Philadelphia: Saunders; 2007. p. 392–418.

5. Ramos GA, Ylagan MV, Romine LE, et al. Diagnostic evaluation of the fetal face using 3-dimensional ultra-sound. Ultrasound Q 2008;24(4):215–23.

6. Campbell S, Lees C, Moscoso G, et al. Ultrasound antenatal diagnosis of cleft palate by a new tech-nique: the 3D "reverse face" view. Ultrasound Ob-stet Gynecol 2005;25(1):12–8.

7. Campbell S, Lees CC. The three-dimensional reverse face (3D RF) view for the diagnosis of cleft palate. Ultrasound Obstet Gynecol 2003;22(5):552–4.

8. Platt LD, Devore GR, Pretorius DH. Improving cleft palate/cleft lip antenatal diagnosis by 3-dimensional sonography: the "flipped face" view. J Ultrasound Med 2006;25(11):1423–30.

9. Benoit B, Chaoui R. Three-dimensional ultrasound with maximal mode rendering: a novel technique for the diagnosis of bilateral or unilateral absence or hypoplasia of nasal bones in second-trimester screening for Down syndrome. Ultrasound Obstet Gynecol 2005;25(1):19–24.

10. Chaoui R, Levaillant JM, Benoit B, et al. Three-dimen-sional sonographic description of abnormal metopic suture in second- and third-trimester fetuses. Ultra-sound Obstet Gynecol 2005;26(7):761–4.

11. Faro C, Benoit B, Wegrzyn P, et al. Three-dimen-sional sonographic description of the fetal frontal bones and metopic suture. Ultrasound Obstet Gyne-col 2005;26(6):618–21.

12. Chang CH, Chang FM, Yu CH, et al. Fetal ear assessment and prenatal detection of aneuploidy by the quantitative three-dimensional ultrasonog-raphy. Ultrasound Med Biol 2000;26(5):743–9.

13. Goncalves LF, Espinoza J, Lee W, et al. Phenotypic characteristics of absent and hypoplastic nasal bones in fetuses with Down syndrome: description by 3-dimensional ultrasonography and clinical signif-icance. J Ultrasound Med 2004;23(12):1619–27.

14. Bianchi DW, Crombleholme TM, D'Alton ME. Fetology: diagnosis and management of the fetal patient. 2nd edition. New York: McGraw-Hill Profes-sional; 2010. p. 221.

15. Matsui H, Hayasaka S, Setogawa T. Congenital cataract in the right eye and primary clinical anophthalmos of the left eye in a patient with cere-bellar hypoplasia. Ann Ophthalmol 1993;25(8): 315–8.

16. Nyberg DA. Diagnostic imaging of fetal anomalies. 2nd edition. Philadelphia: Lippincott Williams & Wilkins; 2002. p. 896.

17. Verma AS, Fitzpatrick DR. Anophthalmia and micro-phthalmia. Orphanet J Rare Dis 2007;2:47.

18. Blazer S, Zimmer EZ, Mezer E, et al. Early and late onset fetal microphthalmia. Am J Obstet Gynecol 2006;194(5):1354–9.

19. Jeanty P, Dramaix-Wilmet M, Van Gansbeke D, et al. Fetal ocular biometry by ultrasound. Radiology 1982;143(2):513–6.

20. Mayden KL, Tortora M, Berkowitz RL, et al. Orbital diameters: a new parameter for prenatal diagnosis and dating. Am J Obstet Gynecol 1982;144(3):289–97.

21. Stoll C, Alembik Y, Dott B, et al. Epidemiology of congenital eye malformations in 131,760 consecu-tive births. Ophthalmic Paediatr Genet 1992;13(3): 179–86.

22. Dekaban AS. Abnormalities in children exposed to x-radiation during various stages of gestation: tenta-tive timetable of radiation injury to the human fetus. I. J Nucl Med 1968;9(9):471–7.

23. Menashe Y, Ben Baruch G, Rabinovitch O, et al. Exophthalmus–prenatal ultrasonic features for diag-nosis of Crouzon syndrome. Prenat Diagn 1989; 9(11):805–8.

24. Miller C, Losken HW, Towbin R, et al. Ultrasound diag-nosis of craniosynostosis. Cleft Palate Craniofac J 2002;39(1):73–80.

25. Hill LM, Thomas ML, Peterson CS. The ultrasonic detection of Apert syndrome. J Ultrasound Med 1987;6(10):601–4.

26. Kaufmann K, Baldinger S, Pratt L. Ultrasound detec-tion of Apert syndrome: a case report and literature review. Am J Perinatol 1997;14(7):427–30.

27. Polin RA, Spitzer AR. Fetal and neonatal secrets. Philadelphia: Hanley & Belfus; 2001. p. 103–4.

28. Stevenson RE. Human malformations and related anomalies. 2nd edition. Oxford (UK): Oxford Univer-sity Press; 2006. p. 323–5.

29. Bronshtein M. Transvaginal sonography of the normal and abnormal fetus. London (UK): Informa Healthcare; 2001. p. 65.

30. Merz E. Ultrasound in obstetrics and gynecology. 2nd revised edition. Stuttgart (NY): Thieme Medical Publishers; 2004. p. 235.

31. Twining P, McHugo JM, Pilling DW. Textbook of fetal abnormalities. Philadelphia: Churchill Livingstone; 2006. p. 384.

32. Vinken PJ, Bruyn GW, Cleovoulou MN. Malforma-tions. Amsterdam (Netherlands): Elsevier Science; 1987. p. 225–42.

33. Sepulveda W, Dezerega V, Be C. First-trimester so-nographic diagnosis of holoprosencephaly: value of the "butterfly" sign. J Ultrasound Med 2004; 23(6):761–5 [quiz: 766–7].

34. Cho FN, Kan YY, Chen SN, et al. Prenatal diagnosis of cyclopia and proboscis in a fetus with normal chromosome at 13 weeks of gestation by three-dimensional transabdominal sonography. Prenat Di-agn 2005;25(11):1059–60.

35. Hsu TY, Chang SY, Ou CY, et al. First trimester diag-nosis of holoprosencephaly and cyclopia with triploidy by transvaginal three-dimensional ultrasonography. Eur J Obstet Gynecol Reprod Biol 2001;96(2):235–7.

36. Tan ST, Mulliken JB. Hypertelorism: nosologic analysis of 90 patients. Plast Reconstr Surg 1997; 99(2):317–27.
37. Kean J, Al-Busaidi SS, Quaba AA. A case report of frontonasal dysplasia. Int J Pediatr Otorhinolaryngol 2010;74(3):306–8.
38. Wieland I, Weidner C, Ciccone R, et al. Contiguous gene deletions involving EFNB1, OPHN1, PJA1 and EDA in patients with craniofrontonasal syndrome. Clin Genet 2007;72(6):506–16.
39. Awwad JT, Azar GB, Karam KS, et al. Ear length: a potential sonographic marker for Down syndrome. Int J Gynaecol Obstet 1994;44(3):233–8.
40. Lettieri L, Rodis JF, Vintzileos AM, et al. Ear length in second-trimester aneuploid fetuses. Obstet Gynecol 1993;81(1):57–60.
41. Hsu TY, Hsu JJ, Chang SY, et al. Prenatal three-dimensional sonographic images associated with Treacher Collins syndrome. Ultrasound Obstet Gynecol 2002;19(4):413–22.
42. Ruangvutilert P, Sutantawibul A, Sunsaneevithayakul P, et al. Ultrasonographic prenatal diagnosis of Treacher Collins syndrome: a case report. J Med Assoc Thai 2003;86(5):482–8.
43. Saraceno J, Lopes T, Pinheiro RH, et al. [Fraser syndrome: case report]. Arq Bras Oftalmol 2008; 71(2):269–72 [in Portuguese].
44. Sharony R, Kidron D, Amiel A, et al. Familial lethal skeletal dysplasia with cloverleaf skull and multiple anomalies of brain, eye, face and heart: a new autosomal recessive multiple congenital anomalies syndrome. Clin Genet 2002;61(5):369–74.
45. Sivan E, Chan L, Uerpairojkit B, et al. Growth of the fetal forehead and normative dimensions developed by three-dimensional ultrasonographic technology. J Ultrasound Med 1997;16(6):401–5.
46. Cicero S, Avgidou K, Rembouskos G, et al. Nasal bone in first-trimester screening for trisomy 21. Am J Obstet Gynecol 2006;195(1):109–14.
47. Kagan KO, Cicero S, Staboulidou I, et al. Fetal nasal bone in screening for trisomies 21, 18 and 13 and Turner syndrome at 11–13 weeks of gestation. Ultrasound Obstet Gynecol 2009; 33(3):259–64.
48. Tardiff A. Dacryocystocele. Available at: http://www.thefetus.net/page.php?id=204. Accessed March 17, 2009.
49. Lembet A, Bodur H, Selam B, et al. Prenatal two- and three-dimensional sonographic diagnosis of dacryocystocele. Prenat Diagn 2008;28(6):554–5.
50. Petrikovsky BM, Kaplan GP. Fetal dacryocystocele: comparing 2D and 3D imaging. Pediatr Radiol 2003;33(8):582–3.
51. Sepulveda W, Wojakowski AB, Elias D, et al. Congenital dacryocystocele: prenatal 2- and 3-dimensional sonographic findings. J Ultrasound Med 2005;24(2):225–30.
52. Nyberg DA, Sickler GK, Hegge FN, et al. Fetal cleft lip with and without cleft palate: US classification and correlation with outcome. Radiology 1995; 195(3):677–84.
53. Berge SJ, Plath H, von Lindern JJ, et al. Natural history of 70 fetuses with a prenatally diagnosed orofacial cleft. Fetal Diagn Ther 2002;17(4):247–51.
54. Genisca AE, Frias JL, Broussard CS, et al. Orofacial clefts in the National Birth Defects Prevention Study, 1997–2004. Am J Med Genet A 2009; 149(6):1149–58.
55. Nyberg DA, Mahony BS, Kramer D. Paranasal echogenic mass: sonographic sign of bilateral complete cleft lip and palate before 20 menstrual weeks. Radiology 1992;184(3):757–9.
56. Bundy AL, Saltzman DH, Emerson D, et al. Sonographic features associated with cleft palate. J Clin Ultrasound 1986;14(6):486–9.
57. Perrotin F, Lardy H, Marret H, et al. [Problems posed by the diagnosis and prenatal management of facial clefts]. Rev Stomatol Chir Maxillofac 2001;102(3/4): 143–52 [in French].
58. Aubry MC, Aubry JP. Prenatal diagnosis of cleft palate: contribution of color Doppler ultrasound. Ultrasound Obstet Gynecol 1992;2(3):221–4.
59. Tolarova MM, Cervenka J. Classification and birth prevalence of orofacial clefts. Am J Med Genet 1998;75(2):126–37.
60. Achiron R, Ben Arie A, Gabbay U, et al. Development of the fetal tongue between 14 and 26 weeks of gestation: in utero ultrasonographic measurements. Ultrasound Obstet Gynecol 1997; 9(1):39–41.
61. Bronshtein M, Zimmer EZ, Tzidony D, et al. Transvaginal sonographic measurement of fetal lingual width in early pregnancy. Prenat Diagn 1998;18(6): 577–80.
62. Mernagh JR, Mohide PT, Lappalainen RE, et al. US assessment of the fetal head and neck: a state-of-the-art pictorial review. Radiographics 1999; 19(Spec No):S229–41.
63. Bianchi DW. Fetology: diagnosis & management of the fetal patient. New York: McGraw-Hill Professional; 2000. p. 1081.
64. Paladini D, Morra T, Guida F, et al. Prenatal diagnosis and perinatal management of a lingual lymphangioma. Ultrasound Obstet Gynecol 1998; 11(2):141–3.
65. Chiang YC, Shih JC, Peng SS, et al. Tongue teratoma–a rare form of fetal extragonadal teratoma diagnosed at 30 weeks' gestation. Ultrasound Obstet Gynecol 2006;28(5):737–41.
66. Bronshtein M, Blazer S, Zalel Y, et al. Ultrasonographic diagnosis of glossoptosis in fetuses with Pierre Robin sequence in early and mid pregnancy. Am J Obstet Gynecol 2005;193(4): 1561–4.

67. Teoh M, Meagher S. First-trimester diagnosis of micrognathia as a presentation of Pierre Robin syndrome. Ultrasound Obstet Gynecol 2003;21(6): 616–8.

68. Rotten D, Levaillant JM, Martinez H, et al. The fetal mandible: a 2D and 3D sonographic approach to the diagnosis of retrognathia and micrognathia. Ultrasound Obstet Gynecol 2002;19(2):122–30.

69. Borenstein M, Persico N, Strobl I, et al. Frontomaxillary and mandibulomaxillary facial angles at 11 + 0 to 13 + 6 weeks in fetuses with trisomy 18. Ultrasound Obstet Gynecol 2007;30(7):928–33.

70. Palit G, Jacquemyn Y, Kerremans M. An objective measurement to diagnose micrognathia on prenatal ultrasound. Clin Exp Obstet Gynecol 2008;35(2): 121–3.

71. Clement K, Chamberlain P, Boyd P, et al. Prenatal diagnosis of an epignathus: a case report and review of the literature. Ultrasound Obstet Gynecol 2001;18(2):178–81.

72. Smith NM, Chambers SE, Billson VR, et al. Oral teratoma (epignathus) with intracranial extension: a report of two cases. Prenat Diagn 1993;13(10):945–52.

73. Midrio P, Grismondi G, Meneghini L, et al. [The EX-utero Intrapartum Technique (EXIT) procedure in Italy]. Minerva Ginecol 2001;53(3):209–14 [in Italian].

74. Mueller DT, Callanan VP. Congenital malformations of the oral cavity. Otolaryngol Clin North Am 2007; 40(1):141–60, vii.

75. Morgan WE, Jones JK, Flaitz CM, et al. Congenital heterotopic gastrointestinal cyst of the oral cavity in a neonate: case report and review of literature. Int J Pediatr Otorhinolaryngol 1996;36(1):69–77.

76. Onderoglu L, Saygan-Karamursel B, Deren O, et al. Prenatal diagnosis of ranula at 21 weeks of gestation. Ultrasound Obstet Gynecol 2003;22(4):399–401.

Imaging of Musculoskeletal Abnormalities with 3-Dimensional Ultrasonography, CT, and MR Imaging

Carlos Cuevas, MD*, Manjiri Dighe, MD

KEYWORDS

- Skeletal dysplasia • Three-dimensional ultrasonography
- Computed tomography • Magnetic resonance imaging

Musculoskeletal (MSK) anomalies are a group of anatomic malformations that may present as an isolated finding or as a part of complex clinical syndromes with multiple findings. These anomalies comprise a group of more than 350 disorders, only approximately 50 of which can be diagnosed prenatally.[1,2] Many of the prenatal-onset skeletal dysplasias are associated with lethality because of pulmonary insufficiency or concomitant visceral abnormalities.[3] The assessment of the extremities and spine could be difficult and may have low sensitivity compared with traditional 2-dimensional (2D) ultrasound examinations.[1,2] It seems necessary to approach the problem with different techniques or modalities that most of the time may increase the accuracy of the diagnosis of significant consequences for the mother and child. In this article the authors review the use of different techniques and compare them with the most traditional 2D ultrasonography examination of the fetus, including 3-dimensional (3D) ultrasonography, and computed tomography (CT) and magnetic resonance (MR) imaging.

Historically, in utero radiographs of a fetus suspected to have skeletal dysplasia were used to confirm ultrasound findings (**Fig. 1**). With marked improvements in ultrasound imaging in the last 10 years, there is little value to this method. Routine ultrasonography is the main screening modality for skeletal disorders, and is also used for counseling regarding optimal patient management (both fetal and maternal) in these cases. Accuracy of conventional ultrasonography, however, for the diagnosis of skeletal dysplasia is only about 65%, because of the complexity and large variety of these diseases.[4,5] Due to the complexity of diagnosis, an organized and comprehensive examination is needed. At the authors' institution a worksheet is used for the same, which includes the routine measurements as well as the 3D datasets.

ULTRASONOGRAPHY

3D ultrasonography has emerged as a technological breakthrough that may significantly increase the diagnostic accuracy of MSK anomalies if used appropriately. It is logical to expect initially some resistance to the introduction of this new technique due to its learning curve, but it is likely that in the near future all the studies will include the use of 3D technology for skeletal assessment because of the multiple benefits expected.[6]

Department of Radiology, University of Washington, 1959 NE Pacific Street, Box 357115, Seattle, WA 98195, USA
* Corresponding author.
E-mail address: sawaller@u.washington.edu

Ultrasound Clin 6 (2011) 39–46
doi:10.1016/j.cult.2011.01.002
1556-858X/11/$ – see front matter © 2011 Published by Elsevier Inc.

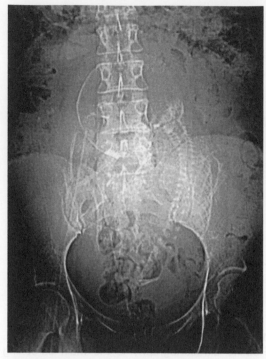

Fig. 1. Radiograph of a pregnant patient. The fetal bony structures are easily visualized, though obscured by the overlying maternal bowel gas and bony structures.

Conventional 2D ultrasonography consists of a tomographic gray-scale image of the subject anatomy. The information displayed in these images corresponds to a single plane in space (per frame). 3D ultrasonography mode consists of a collection of data from a defined volume. This 3D dataset can be displayed as multiplanar

mode: multiple tomographic images reconstructed in any plane of the space acquired (**Fig. 2**). Because the data acquired is always asymmetric (ie, anisotropic voxel), every deviation from the originally acquired plane is associated with a loss of image quality. Other possible displays include 3D volume-rendering models, including surface and maximum rendering (**Fig. 3**).[7]

Most of the commercially available high-end ultrasound scanners have the capability of acquiring, storing, and processing a 3D dataset. 3D datasets can be acquired in 3 different ways: using conventional ultrasonography and acquiring free-hand sweep, mechanically powered 3D transducers, or electronic array transducers. A conventional ultrasound transducer could be used to obtain 3D data, in which case the sonographer has to perform the sweep manually. Mechanically powered transducers are also available. These transducers are capable of performing one or multiple sweeps while being held steady over the region of interest, due to the built-in mechanism that produces motion of the crystals. Four-dimensional (4D) movies can be obtained with these transducers while acquiring multiple continuous sweeps. Kurjak and colleagues[8] found in their study that the key benefit of 4D ultrasonography was in visualization of details regarding the dynamics of small anatomic structures. Therefore, body and limb movements could be visualized earlier than with 2D data. Another kind of transducer available has an electronic array of crystals, and when fired electronically can acquire isotropic 3D data that can be reformatted in any plane.

The dataset can be processed in the ultrasound machine instantly to prepare the images that will

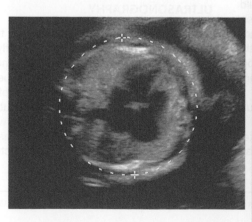

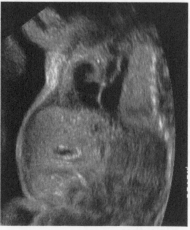

Fig. 2. Transverse image through the fetal chest. Chest circumference measured 20 cm, which was at 25th% tile for this 28 week-old fetus. Coronal reformat through the fetal chest and abdomen acquired from a 3D dataset shows the discrepancy between the size of the fetal chest and the abdomen, suggesting smaller than normal chest.

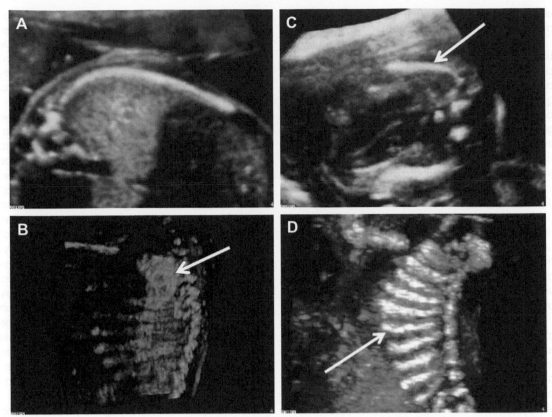

Fig. 3. Fetal ribs. (*A*) Transverse ultrasound image through the fetal chest and (*B*) 3D reformat; note that the rib covers greater than two-thirds of the circumference of the chest wall. Fetal scapula is also seen on the 3D reformat (*arrow*). (*C*) Fetus with short rib polydactyly showing small ribs bilaterally (*arrow*); note that the ribs in this fetus do not cover greater than 50% of the circumference of the chest wall. (*D*) 3D reformat of the chest shows the smaller size of the ribs (*arrow*).

be sent to PACS (Picture Archiving and Communication System), or the whole volume of data sent to a remote work station in the reading room where the sonologist can process the data for interpretation and storage. Surface-rendering images can be reconstructed easily if the structures are surrounded by abundant anechoic fluid; this clean interface between fluid and soft tissue generates sharp images (**Fig. 4**). If the anatomic structures were in direct contact with other parts of the anatomy it would be necessary to use the electronic scalpel for trimming part of the volume, to obtain a clear view of the extremity of interest. To decrease the occurrence of motion artifacts it

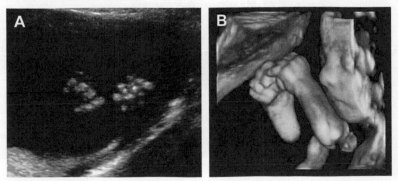

Fig. 4. Clean interface with fluid in this fetus with known trisomy 18 and polyhydramnios shows clenched fists on B-mode ultrasonography (*A*) and on a 3D reformat (*B*).

is recommended to acquire the dataset while the patients are holding their breath.

Although the 3D technique can be used at any time during pregnancy, the ideal conditions for performing fetal 3D skeletal studies need to balance a relatively large fetus (ie, advanced gestational age) with good fluid/fetal size ratio. In practical terms this corresponds to 20 to 30 weeks gestational age, and is particularly true for the assessment of the hands and feet.[9] The best position for the fetus is with the extremities facing the transducer, perpendicular to the ultrasound beam.

The benefit of using 3D ultrasonography for the assessment of the extremities is a more accurate diagnosis of the pathology and better demonstration of normal findings. This improvement is particularly true for more complex structures such as hands or feet,[9–11] and possibly less significant for proximal limbs unless the condition to be assessed produces typically complex fixed positions of the extremities (**Figs. 5** and **6**).

The existence of a learning curve for the performance of a 3D fetal ultrasonogram is unquestionable, and it seems logical that with increasing experience of the team the acquisition of volumes of data and the operation of the 3D workstation will become more efficient. However, there remains still the question over the time required to perform and read 3D versus 2D ultrasonography. Benacerraf and colleagues[12] suggested in a recent study that a 3D-only protocol may save time compared with a 2D protocol, but the same investigators in a follow-up article suggest that a quick 3D-only acquisition may also decrease detection of fetal anomalies including MSK malformations.[6] A 3D-only protocol is not yet sufficient for routine use, and for every kind of malformation at any gestational age some balance must be found between

2D and the use of the new 3D technology. Elaborated postprocessing of the images is only necessary in complex diagnosis, which would involve only a small number of patients. However, surface-rendering images accelerate and simplify the discussion of complex cases with the referring clinicians as well as with the patients.[7]

One of the limitations of the equipment is the capability of managing large amounts of data, because some 3D studies may accumulate 1 to 4 gigabytes of information depending on the protocol and postprocessing of images. However, this is now less of an issue with the increasing computing power and larger sizes of the onboard storage capacity of the ultrasound machines. The official document from the American Institute of Ultrasound in Medicine states that "currently, 2-dimensional (2D) gray-scale real-time sonography is the primary method of medically indicated anatomic imaging with ultrasound. The 2D display remains the primary method of image presentation regardless of the method of acquisition. While 3D ultrasound may be helpful in diagnosis, it is currently an adjunct to, but not a replacement for, 2D ultrasound. As with any developing technology, its clinical value may improve and its diagnostic role will be periodically reevaluated."

Sensitivity of 3D ultrasonography for detecting anomalies in the extremities was 96.3% versus 48.2% for 2D ultrasonography in a study of 26 fetuses with trisomy 18.[11] In the same study, all the other organ system anomalies showed just mild differences between the two modalities. Ploekinger-Ulm and colleagues[9] showed that 3D ultrasonography was superior to 2D ultrasonography in visualizing the fetal hand at any stage of pregnancy. Kos and colleagues[13] found in their study that the positive predictive value for 2D

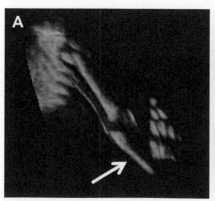
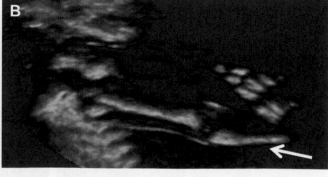

Fig. 5. B-mode image (*A*) and a 3D reformat (*B*) through the fetal arm shows flexion of the hand with absence of the radius and smaller than normal size of the ulna (*arrow*).

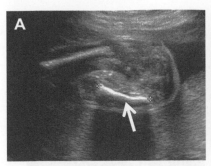 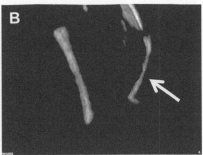

Fig. 6. Fetus with proximal focal femoral deficiency. B-mode (*A*) and 3D reformat images (*B*) show smaller size of the left femur (*arrow*) compared with the right femur. This suggests proximal focal femoral deficiency.

sonography in the detection of clubfoot was considerably lower (67.8%) than that of 3D sonography (89.9%). These investigators recommend surface-mode imaging as the best technique for recognizing surface anatomy, integrity of skin cover, and topographic relationships between the segments of each limb. Surface rendering of the suspected anomalous limb seemed to be the most efficient modality in the diagnosis of angular deformation and joint contractures. Unfortunately, without amniotic fluid surrounding the limb surface, rendering was less effective in their study. 3D examination of the fetal hand and foot allowed them to obtain simultaneous evaluation in 3 orthogonal planes with a single volume acquisition.

Krakow and colleagues,[14] in their limited study of 5 fetuses including one patient each with thanatophoric dysplasia, achondrogenesis II/hypochondrogenesis, achondroplasia, chondrodysplasia punctata (rhizomelic form), and Apert syndrome, found that for all 5 fetuses the correct diagnosis was made by analysis of the 2D images. In each case the 3D images confirmed the preliminary diagnosis, and for many findings it improved the visualization of the abnormalities.

A study[15] involving only fetuses with thanatophoric dysplasia (TD) found that 3D ultrasonography can detect fetal TD and provide additional vivid illustration after various modes of reconstruction that 2D sonography cannot afford. 3D sonography may contribute significantly to the detection of TD in utero and provide a novel visual depiction of this defect after reconstruction. The investigators concluded that 3D sonography may help in prenatal diagnosis as well as consultation with referring physicians.[15]

COMPUTED TOMOGRAPHY

CT uses x-rays to generate medical images, therefore the technical aspects of the examination are

of main importance in order to comply with the As Low As Reasonably Achievable (ALARA) principles concerning radiation dose. There are several technical advances now available that can help to decrease the radiation dose in a CT study, including: more efficient detectors, ASIR (Adaptive Statistical Iterative Reconstruction) and other new reconstruction algorithms using iterative reconstruction techniques instead of the traditional filtered back-projection (FBP), x-ray filters, and tube current modulation programs. Sixty-four-slice multidetector CTs and other modern CT scanners are capable of obtaining an isotropic volume of data; this means that the images can be reconstructed in any plane of the space with the same resolution. This approach is particularly useful for adequate display of the fetal tomographic images and comparison with other techniques such as ultrasonography or MR imaging (**Fig. 7**). To avoid motion artifacts, the temporal resolution has to be maximized using the highest rotation speed possible and a pitch of 1 or 1.3. With the use of a workstation, a 3D rendered model of the ossified skeleton is quick and easy to obtain.

Ultrasound visualization of the fetal skeleton is limited, and CT may be useful in evaluation of fetal skeletal dysplasias as suggested by some prior studies. In their study, Ruano and colleagues[16] reported 3 cases of achondroplasia, 2 cases of osteogenesis imperfecta type II, and 1 case of chondrodysplasia punctata diagnosed by CT. 2D ultrasonography made the correct diagnosis in 4 cases. 3D helical CT (HCT) achieved an accurate diagnosis in all 6 cases. A case report by Tsutsumi and colleagues[17] of a fetus with TD demonstrated a greater number of findings on CT than on ultrasonography. In their study of 10 fetuses with some form of dysplasia, Cassart and colleagues[18] found that 2D ultrasonography provided the correct diagnosis in only 2 of the 11 cases. CT yielded the correct diagnosis in 8 cases. 3D CT

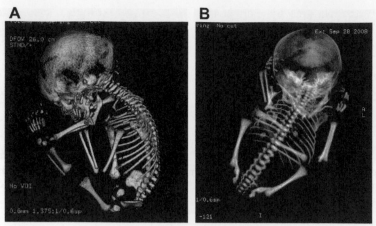

Fig. 7. 3D reformat (A) from a fetal CT performed for a maternal indication. Note the clear visualization of the fetal structures. A MIP reformat (B) shows a pseudo-radiograph appearance.

was more accurate than 2D ultrasonography in visualizing vertebral anomalies, pelvic bone malformations, and enlarged metaphysis or synostoses in long bones. Hence there are certain clinical situations, particularly in the evaluation of musculoskeletal dysplasias, where CT scanning has been shown to provide added value.

MAGNETIC RESONANCE IMAGING

Most of the fetal MR images are obtained in single-shot T2-weighted images (half Fourier acquisition single-shot turbo spin echo [HASTE], single-shot fast spin echo [SSFSE]) that are very fast and have a minimal amount of artifacts. The key is to

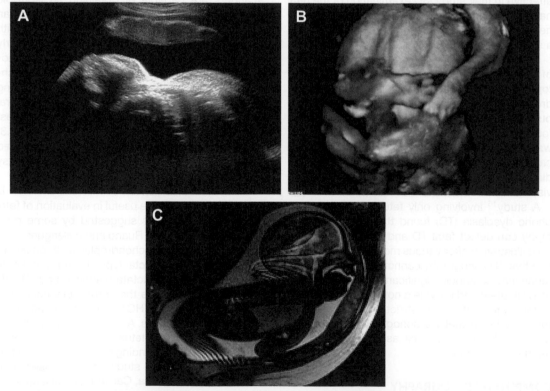

Fig. 8. Fetus with arthrogryposis. Sagittal B-mode image (A) through the fetal neck showed persistent hyperflexion of the fetal neck. 3D reformat (B) shows persistent flexion of the arms with a crossed appearance. Sagittal image from fetal MR imaging (C) shows persistent hyperflexion of the neck.

obtain adequate alignment with the part of the skeleton that is being studied, which can be challenging in some cases of very active fetuses or easier in cases with pathologic features associated with decreased motion.

MR imaging has the potential to identify features of epiphyseal, physeal, metaphyseal, and cortical development. Connolly and colleagues,[19] in their study on pig fetuses, found that MR imaging enabled visualization of maturational changes in the fetal pig skeleton that were previously demonstrable primarily at histologic analysis. These investigators suggest that MR imaging evaluation of these changes may be useful in improving the determination of gestational age, evaluating fetal maturity, and enabling the early detection of focal or generalized abnormalities of the fetal skeleton. Although current technologies do not enable the visualization of these structures in vivo, in the future optimized MR imaging techniques may enable the detection of these structures in fetuses. Echo-planar imaging sequences can mainly be used to image fetal bone and can be used to obtain an overview of thoracic size and skeletal development. MR imaging has the advantage of comprehensively displaying the fetal body, including the dependent side that is relatively inaccessible sonographically. However, MR imaging may not capture both hands and feet, due to fetal movement. This restriction can be overcome by using dynamic thick-slab steady-state free precession sequences. The authors have performed fetal MR imaging primarily for fetal arthrogryposis to assess the fetal head position and the amount of extension, which is useful for planning the delivery of these fetuses (**Fig. 8**).

In a study comparing MR imaging with 3D ultrasonography the authors obtained concordant findings, with the advantage of fetal movement assessment that can be done only with ultrasonography.[20]

SUMMARY

2D ultrasonography has been used traditionally as the main imaging modality for the study of all fetal anomalies, but it can be limited in the assessment of some cases of musculoskeletal pathology. The selective use of complementary imaging modalities can significantly improve the detection and characterization of skeletal anomalies in the fetus. 3D ultrasonography can be used in a wide range of anatomic abnormalities, but seems to provide a significant advantage over 2D ultrasonography for the study of fetal hands and feet. The use of CT in fetal images is generally limited due to the problem of radiation exposure, but CT should be

considered for the analysis of skeletal dysplasias where it can provide extraordinarily good quality images of the entire skeleton. MR imaging is a safe modality that can provide useful additional information for complex fetal syndromes that involve multiple organ systems, especially when the central nervous system is involved. Each modality has advantages and limitations that should be considered on an individual case basis, but institutional guidelines can be useful in the decision-making process.

REFERENCES

1. Superti-Furga A, Bonafé L, Rimoin DL. Molecular-pathogenetic classification of genetic disorders of the skeleton. Am J Med Genet 2001;106:282–93.
2. Hall CM. International nosology and classification of constitutional disorders of bone (2001). Am J Med Genet 2002;113:65–77.
3. Lachman R, Taybi H. Taybi and Lachman's radiology of syndromes, metabolic disorders and skeletal dysplasias. Philadelphia: Mosby Elsevier; 2006.
4. Doray B, Favre R, Viville B, et al. Prenatal sonographic diagnosis of skeletal dysplasias. A report of 47 cases. Ann Genet 2000;43:163–9.
5. Parilla BV, Leeth EA, Kambich MP, et al. Antenatal detection of skeletal dysplasias. J Ultrasound Med 2003;22:255–8 [quiz: 259–61].
6. Benacerraf BR. Tomographic sonography of the fetus: is it accurate enough to be a frontline screen for fetal malformation? J Ultrasound Med 2006;25:687–9.
7. Dückelmann AM, Kalache KD. Three-dimensional ultrasound in evaluating the fetus. Prenat Diagn 2010;30:631–8.
8. Kurjak A, Vecek N, Hafner T, et al. Prenatal diagnosis: what does four-dimensional ultrasound add? J Perinat Med 2002;30:57–62.
9. Ploeckinger-Ulm B, Ulm MR, Lee A, et al. Antenatal depiction of fetal digits with three-dimensional ultrasonography. Am J Obstet Gynecol 1996;175:571–4.
10. Rypens F, Dubois J, Garel L, et al. Obstetric US: watch the fetal hands. Radiographics 2006;26: 811–29 [discussion: 830–1].
11. Zheng Y, Zhou XD, Zhu YL, et al. Three- and 4-dimensional ultrasonography in the prenatal evaluation of fetal anomalies associated with trisomy 18. J Ultrasound Med 2008;27:1041–51.
12. Benacerraf BR, Shipp TD, Bromley B. How sonographic tomography will change the face of obstetric sonography: a pilot study. J Ultrasound Med 2005;24:371–8.
13. Kos M, Hafner T, Funduk-Kurjak B, et al. Limb deformities and three-dimensional ultrasound. J Perinat Med 2002;30:40–7.
14. Krakow D, Williams J, Poehl M, et al. Use of three-dimensional ultrasound imaging in the diagnosis of

prenatal-onset skeletal dysplasias. Ultrasound Obstet Gynecol 2003;21:467–72.

15. Tsai PY, Chang CH, Yu CH, et al. Thanatophoric dysplasia: role of 3-dimensional sonography. J Clin Ultrasound 2009;37:31–4.

16. Ruano R, Molho M, Roume J, et al. Prenatal diagnosis of fetal skeletal dysplasias by combining two-dimensional and three-dimensional ultrasound and intrauterine three-dimensional helical computer tomography. Ultrasound Obstet Gynecol 2004;24:134–40.

17. Tsutsumi S, Sawai H, Nishimura G, et al. Prenatal diagnosis of thanatophoric dysplasia by 3-D helical computed tomography and genetic analysis. Fetal Diagn Ther 2008;24:420–4.

18. Cassart M, Massez A, Cos T, et al. Contribution of three-dimensional computed tomography in the assessment of fetal skeletal dysplasia. Ultrasound Obstet Gynecol 2007;29:537–43.

19. Connolly SA, Jaramillo D, Hong JK, et al. Skeletal development in fetal pig specimens: MR imaging of femur with histologic comparison. Radiology 2004;233:505–14.

20. Behairy NH, Talaat S, Saleem SN, et al. Magnetic resonance imaging in fetal anomalies: what does it add to 3D and 4D US? Eur J Radiol 2010;74:250–5.

Advances in Fetal Cardiac Imaging

Margaret M. Vernon, MD*, Mark B. Lewin, MD

KEYWORDS
- Fetal • Echocardiogram • Prenatal • Ultrasound • Cardiac

Imaging the fetal heart has evolved considerably since the first report of ultrasonographic visualization of the fetal heart in the early 1970s. From that description of ventricular output inferred from m-mode tracings,[1] one can trace the roots of fetal echocardiography. This article reviews the current state of the art in ultrasonographic evaluation of the fetal cardiovascular system.

Ultrasound remains the primary imaging modality for evaluating the fetal heart and cardiovascular system. Beginning in the 1980s, commonly used transthoracic cross-sectional views of the heart had been reproduced in utero,[2] and the possibility of prenatal detection of major congenital heart disease was realized. As in utero ultrasonographic evaluations became mainstream, the goal of in utero identification of congenital heart disease was established.

Today, fetal cardiac imaging has moved from a novel, reportable technique to a component of the nearly universal mid-trimester fetal anatomic survey. In addition, a comprehensive ultrasonographic evaluation of the fetal cardiovascular system, the fetal echocardiogram, has emerged. As part of the mid-trimester screening ultrasound, a 4-chamber view of the heart is obtained, and if possible, views of both outflow tracts. Abnormal or unsatisfactory (the inability to establish normal) cardiac views obtained as part of this survey account for more than 20% of all referrals for fetal echocardiography and lead to over half of all prenatal diagnoses of congenital heart disease. The role of routine obstetric ultrasound screening is critical in the prenatal identification of congenital heart disease.

Alternatively, it is well established that a variety of maternal or fetal disorders may place a fetus at increased risk for congenital heart disease (**Table 1**). In these circumstances, a fetal echocardiogram is recommended as well. Of these indications, a positive family history accounts for another nearly 20% of referrals for fetal echocardiography, though leading to the identification of fewer than 5% of all prenatal diagnoses. All combined, in about 5% of all pregnancies a fetal echocardiogram is obtained.

TECHNICAL IMPROVEMENTS
Improvements in Image Resolution

Historically the goal of fetal echocardiography was simply to detect congenital heart disease. While this goal remains lofty, as recently as the early 1990s the rate of prenatal diagnosis of congenital heart disease was fewer than 10% of infants undergoing cardiac surgery in the first month of life,[3] hence an emerging goal is to establish an accurate diagnosis. Today detailed anatomic diagnoses can successfully be established with excellent correlation with postnatal echocardiograms. Arriving at an accurate diagnosis depends first, on the ability to obtain a complete set of images and second, on the correct interpretation of those images. The development of high-frequency transducers (6–10 MHz) with variable focus has been instrumental in establishing this goal. Today's ultrasound transducers provide a markedly improved level of image quality compared with that of the 1990s (**Fig. 1**).

The authors have nothing to disclose.
Division of Cardiology, Seattle Children's Hospital, M/S G-0035, PO Box 5371, Seattle, WA 98145, USA
* Corresponding author.
E-mail address: meg.vernon@seattlechildrens.org

Ultrasound Clin 6 (2011) 47–56
doi:10.1016/j.cult.2011.01.007
1556-858X/11/$ – see front matter © 2011 Published by Elsevier Inc.

Table 1
Indications for fetal echocardiography

Maternal Indications	Fetal Indications
Family history of congenital heart disease including prior child or pregnancy with congenital heart disease	Abnormal obstetric screening ultrasonography
Metabolic disorders (eg, diabetes)	Extracardiac abnormality
Exposure to teratogens	Chromosomal abnormality
Exposure to prostaglandin synthetase inhibitors (ibuprofen)	Arrhythmia
Infection (rubella, Coxsackie, parvovirus B19)	Hydrops
Autoimmune diagnosis (eg, Sjögren, systemic lupus erythematosus)	Increased first-trimester nuchal translucency
Familial inherited disorder (Marfan, Noonan)	Multiple gestation and suspicion for twin-twin transfusion syndrome
In vitro fertilization	

Today the identification of arch branching patterns and systemic and pulmonary venous drainage patterns is frequently possible. The entry of the superior and inferior vena cava into the right atrium can be documented in an image identical to the transthoracic bicaval view. The pulmonary veins are often best evaluated in the 4-chamber view. By 2-dimensional (2-D) imaging pulmonary veins can be seen entering the left atrium, which can be confirmed by color Doppler (**Fig. 2**).

Unfortunately, fetal lie and position, maternal body habitus and placental position, oligohydramnios, and the relatively fixed fetal position associated with advanced gestational age or a multiple gestation will always limit the acoustic windows available.

EXAMINATION STANDARDIZATION

Successful fetal cardiac imaging requires the ability to obtain and properly interpret standard views as well as the ability to approach the heart from multiple different orientations given the available acoustic windows.

Screening Cardiac Views

Depending on the population, more than one-third of all cases of congenital heart disease occur in pregnancies not identified as high risk. For this reason, the prenatal detection of congenital heart disease relies most heavily on the images obtained during the nearly universal mid-trimester anatomic scan. In the mid 1990s, the American Institute of

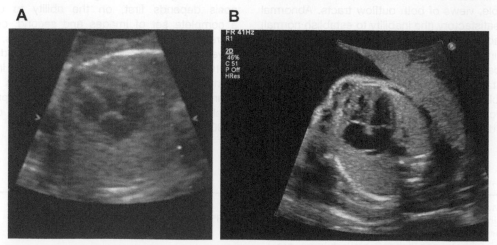

Fig. 1. Four-chamber view from the late 1990s (*A*) compared with one obtained at 20 weeks during the summer of 2010 (*B*).

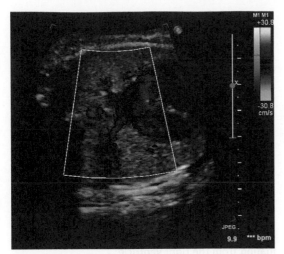

Fig. 2. Pulmonary venous return is seen entering the left atrium from both lung fields.

Ultrasound in Medicine (1994) and the American College of Radiology (1995) incorporated the 4-chamber view into their formal guidelines for the screening fetal ultrasound. This single view is abnormal in up to 60% of fetuses with major congenital heart disease if it is interpreted correctly.[4]

The 4-chamber view is the most important in a comprehensive examination of the fetal heart (Fig. 3 and MMC 1). The 4-chamber view illustrates the pulmonary venous connections, the atrioventricular valves and cardiac crux, the atrial septum, and the inlet and portions of the muscular ventricular septum. It is important to assess for symmetry in size of atria and ventricles. Late in gestation the right ventricle may be slightly larger than the left ventricle. The right ventricle, in its normal position, is posterior to the sternum and identified by the presence of the moderator band. The image is obtained in a transverse scanning plane (cross section). In comparison to transthoracic imaging, the view can be obtained by rotating 90° from a long-axis view of the fetus due to the large size of the fetal liver and more transverse orientation of the fetal heart. The valve leaflets should open fully and should appear thin. Leaflets should show complete coaptation. Presence of the foramenal flap in the left atrium as well as the coronary sinus (Fig. 4) should be apparent.

The 4-chamber view may fail to detect a significant percentage of major, frequently ductal-dependent congenital heart disease (ie, pulmonary atresia, tetralogy of Fallot, double-outlet right ventricle, transposition of the great arteries, and truncus arteriosus).

Many investigators have demonstrated an incremental value of adding outflow tracts to the routine screening fetal ultrasound. In 2007, The American College of Radiology (ACR) Practice Guideline for the Performance of Obstetrical Ultrasound,[5] which has been adopted by the American College of Obstetricians and Gynecologists (ACOG),[6] included a 4-chamber view and, if technically feasible, visualization of both the right and left ventricular the outflow tracts. It is estimated that by combining the 4-chamber and outflow tract views, 75% of all congenital heart lesions could be detected prenatally.

The left ventricular outflow tract (LVOT) can be obtained by rotating the transducer from the

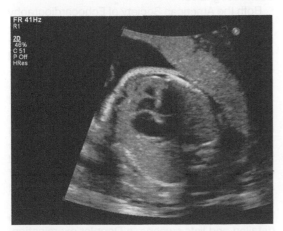

Fig. 3. Four-chamber view of the heart with the atrioventricular valves closed. The moderator band is clearly seen in the right ventricle and the normal very slight apical displacement of the tricuspid valve annulus is noted.

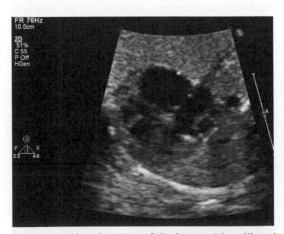

Fig. 4. Four-chamber view of the heart with a dilated coronary sinus noted in the left atrium. Further imaging confirmed the presence of a left-sided superior vena cava.

4-chamber view and angling very slightly toward the fetal right shoulder, a similar movement to the transthoracic imaging in a pediatric patient (**Fig. 5**). Once the LVOT is opened up, rocking the transducer slightly anteriorly (and cranially) will allow visualization of the main pulmonary artery arising from the right ventricle (**Fig. 6**) in normally related great arteries. The main pulmonary artery and ascending aorta should criss-cross (MMC 2). In transposed great arteries, the aorta and pulmonary artery are oriented parallel to each other as the pulmonary artery arises from the left ventricle and courses posteriorly before bifurcating (MMC 3). If the great arteries are not clearly seen crossing, the possibility of a conotruncal malformation, specifically transposition of the great arteries, should be investigated. The outflow tracts can also be evaluated in a short-axis image similar to the pediatric parasternal short axis. In this image, the pulmonary artery is seen wrapping around the aorta, which is visible en face.

Since the addition of the outflow tracts, considerable debate has remained about the inclusion of the words "if possible." This author shares the opinion that establishing the origin of the main pulmonary artery from the right ventricle and the aorta from the left ventricle is mandatory. This being said, the formal incorporation of the 4-chamber view with an attempt at viewing both outflow tracts into the routine screening fetal ultrasound represents an important advance in fetal cardiac imaging.

Components of a Fetal Echocardiogram

The demand for and number of fetal echocardiograms performed has increased drastically over the past decade. Similar to transthoracic imaging, fetal echocardiography depends on the ability to

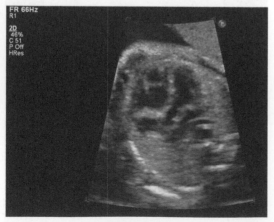

Fig. 5. The left ventricular outflow tract is seen originating from the left ventricle.

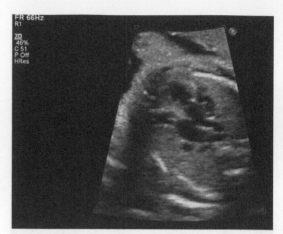

Fig. 6. The right ventricular outflow tract is seen originating from the right ventricle.

obtain standard views and evaluate structures in orthogonal views. In the ideal situation, the echocardiogram is approached in a systematic fashion similar to a postnatal transthoracic examination. This being said, the fetus may be very active, changing position many times during the ultrasound procedure, and the examiner may need to be piece together many partial images to form a composite picture, particularly in the presence of complex congenital heart disease. Frequently these examinations can take well over an hour to complete. In addition, fetal echocardiograms are interpreted by obstetricians, cardiologists, and radiologists and are performed by sonographers working closely with these varied practitioners. Because of this variety, and recognizing the growth in the field, the need to standardize the components of the fetal echocardiogram has been recognized.

Both the American Society of Echocardiography (ASE) (2004)[7] and the American Institute of Ultrasound in Medicine (AIUM) (2010)[8] have published practice guidelines for the performance of the fetal echocardiogram. The AIUM guideline was published in conjunction with the ACOG and the Society for Maternal Fetal Medicine (SMFM), and is endorsed by the ACR. The essential components of a comprehensive evaluation following the ASE Guidelines are listed in **Table 2**. All agree that the performance and interpretation of a fetal echocardiogram requires a unique set of advanced skills because the fetal heart is small and dynamic, and its pathology is limitless. Whereas the ASE Practice Guideline is quite detailed and lists sweeps, a Doppler examination, and measurement data as essential components of the fetal echocardiogram, the AIUM guideline recommends spectral and color Doppler, and measurement of anatomic structures only if there

Table 2
Components of the fetal echocardiogram

Overview	Fetal number and position Stomach position and abdominal situs Cardiac position

Biometric
  examination
	Cardiothoracic ratio
	Biparietal diameter and
	    head circumference
	Femur length
	Abdominal circumference

Cardiac imaging	Four-chamber view
	Left ventricular
	    outflow tract
	Right ventricular
	    outflow tract
	Great arteries
	Three-vessel view
	Bicaval view
	Ductal arch
	Aortic arch

Doppler
  examination
	Inferior and superior
	    vena cava
	Pulmonary veins
	Ductus venosus
	Foramen ovale
	Atrioventricular valves
	Semilunar valves
	Ductus arteriosus
	Transverse aortic arch
	Umbilical artery
	Umbilical vein

Measurement
  data
	Atrioventricular valve
	    diameter
	Semilunar valve diameter
	Main pulmonary artery
	Ascending aorta
	Branch pulmonary arteries
	Transverse aortic arch
	Ventricular length
	Ventricular short-axis
	    dimensions

Examination of
  rate and rhythm
	M-mode of atrial and
	    ventricular wall motion
	Doppler examination of
	    atrial and ventricular
	    flow patterns

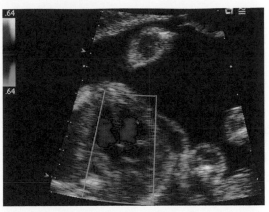

Fig. 7. Four-chamber view with normal color Doppler across the tricuspid and mitral valves during diastolic filling.

very small structures, either because the structure is abnormally small (hypoplastic ascending aorta) or the evaluation is being undertaken early in fetal life (pulmonary venous return).

EARLIER IMAGING

Pregnancy is routinely split into trimesters: conception to 13 weeks, 14 to 26 weeks, and 27 weeks to full term (40 weeks). Historically the advocated optimal timing for performance of a comprehensive transabdominal fetal echocardiography is between 18 and 22 weeks' gestation. At this gestational age, the fetus has grown such that it is out of the maternal pelvis, there are still large pockets of amniotic fluid to be used, and fetal position is still variable. These characteristics combined lead to a complete study in most patients. This procedure has not changed; however, we are moving into an era of early risk assessment and recognition of fetal anomalies. With this has come an interest in earlier evaluation of the fetal heart. Fortunately, technological advances in sonographic instrumentation, specifically the availability of high-resolution probes, have led to earlier attempts at evaluation of the fetal heart.

The first-trimester screen performed between 11 and 13 weeks' gestation combines maternal human chorionic gonadotropin (hCG) and pregnancy-associated plasma protein A (PAPP-A) blood levels as well as fetal nuchal translucency (NT) with maternal age, to come up with a composite risk of a chromosomal abnormality. The NT, the measurement of the thickness of the fluid collection observed beneath the fetal skin along the posterior neck, is increased in fetuses with Down syndrome and other chromosomal

is a suspected abnormality. Color Doppler is extremely useful in fetal cardiac assessment. It can be used to quickly confirm normal flow (**Fig. 7**) or alternatively abnormal flow. Color Doppler evaluation of the aortic and ductal arches showing normal antegrade flow is essential, as flow reversal is consistent with severe congenital heart disease such as semilunar valve hypoplasia or atresia. It is particularly useful in identifying a structure as vascular or during the search for abnormalities. Initially introduced as a noninvasive assessment of increased risk for a chromosomal abnormality, an increased NT has now been identified as a risk factor for congenital heart disease. This increased risk holds in chromosomally normal fetuses.[9,10] Not surprisingly, there has been a surge of interest in earlier diagnosis of congenital heart disease since this was discovered, as it provides invaluable reassurance to the mother with a fetus at high risk for heart disease who has a normal study or, alternatively, provides more time for further testing if heart disease is detected. In addition, earlier diagnosis allows for an earlier, safer, and less traumatic termination if chosen.

Today, transabdominal fetal echocardiography is feasible in the late first and early second trimesters (**Fig. 8**; MMC 4 and 5). In experienced centers, a complete transabdominal evaluation of the fetal heart can reliably be obtained in all patients by 15 weeks' gestation.[11] A limited number of reports describe the utility of transvaginal imaging between 10 and 13 weeks.[12]

As there are some lesions that tend to progress or evolve in utero, primarily outflow tract obstruction, it is strongly recommended that all early fetal echocardiograms be followed by evaluation at mid-gestation. Some defects cannot, however, develop from a normal-looking heart, including transposition of the great arteries, atrioventricular canal defects, double-outlet right ventricle, truncus arteriosus, total anomalous pulmonary venous return, and Ebstein anomaly, and early reassurance is beneficial.

QUANTITATIVE ASSESSMENT

The goal of fetal echocardiography has been to provide a primarily structural, cardiac diagnosis for prenatal counseling. A quantitative assessment of fetal cardiovascular structure and function is increasingly becoming a part of fetal echocardiography.

Normal Data Sets

Serial observation of in utero heart disease has provided critical insight into the evolution of congenital heart disease and potential for in utero progression.[13] Though not all structures require measuring, especially if visually there are no concerns, structures can be measured and compared with established normal subjects for varying gestational ages. Serial assessment has been aided by the compilation of normative data sets. Similar to the normative data sets available for transthoracic echocardiography, the compilation of normative data allows comparison of obtained measurements with established normals.[14,15] The creation of z-scores,[16,17] which quantify the degree to which a given measurement lies above or below the mean value for a given population, have been instrumental to fetal echocardiography and the ability to longitudinally track pathology. Assessment of in utero disease severity is challenging, as many of the well-understood postnatal hemodynamic findings are altered or absent in the presence of the placental circulation. In particular, equalization of pressures between the left and right ventricles and aorta and pulmonary arteries makes evaluation of semilunar valve pathology, known to progress in utero, challenging. Fetal echocardiography relies on the secondary findings for indirect measurement of severity. Critical to the applicability of these data sets is an understanding of how a measurement is obtained and to what it is indexed. In utero measurement sets have been created, which

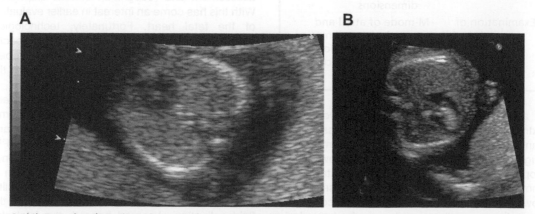

Fig. 8. (*A*) Four-chamber view at 14 weeks' gestation. (*B*) Abnormal early fetal echocardiogram at 16 weeks' gestation. There is severe left ventricular dysfunction, the left ventricular myocardium is bright, and there was minimal flow detectable across the aortic valve consistent with severe aortic stenosis.

index measurements for gestational age as well as biometric measurements (biparietal diameter, head circumference, and femur length).

Access to in utero serial observatory data sets as well as normal data sets has aided the evolving field of in utero cardiac intervention. A relatively limited number of centers have cautiously explored this field in hopes of altering outcome for a few of the most severe and devastating forms of congenital heart disease, including critical aortic[18] and pulmonary stenosis. Early in utero interventional data are encouraging, with normalization of growth and tolerance of biventricular circulation postnatally in some patients uniformly destined for single ventricular palliation.[19]

Composite Comparative Scores

Semiquantitative scoring systems have been created to estimate severity, facilitate serial assessment, and predict outcome. Increasingly these models of standardization of assessment will become important as in utero interventions are introduced in hopes of altering the natural course of a disease state. To date, cardiovascular scores have been developed for fetal heart failure,[20] twin-twin transfusion syndrome, and critical aortic stenosis.

For fetal congestive heart failure, the cardiovascular profile score (CVP)[21] comprises a 10-point scoring system that combines data collected during a fetal echocardiogram known to be associated with perinatal mortality: hydrops, cardiac size, abnormal myocardial function, redistribution of cardiac output, and abnormal venous Doppler patterns. The maximum CVP score is 10 and the minimum is 0. Deductions from the maximum of 1 or 2 points for each of the 5 categories are made for abnormal findings.

Ventricular Function

The evaluation of fetal cardiac function was limited historically to an eyeballed qualitative global assessment of systolic function (good, poor, depressed) with no defined criteria to assure inter-observer reproducibility. As perinatology has moved from quiet observation of high-risk fetuses to in utero management, early induced delivery, and even in utero intervention, an interest in a reproducible quantitative assessment of myocardial function has developed. Evaluation of heart size, heart rate, and the presence or absence of hydrops can provide clues to cardiac function, and indices of systolic and diastolic function are being investigated.

Systolic function

Fetuses with lesions known to effect cardiac function such as volume overload (in the recipient in twin-twin transfusion syndrome), a hyperdynamic circulation (arterio-venous malformation), cardiac compression (diaphragmatic hernia or lung lesions), and increased placental resistance (intrauterine growth restriction and placental insufficiency) have been studied and reported. Systolic function is estimated qualitatively and can also be quantified by calculating the shortening fraction from either 2-D images or M-mode tracings. The simplest calculation is the M-mode derived estimated shortening fraction, calculated as the end-diastolic dimension minus the end-systolic dimension divided by the end-diastolic dimension. One of the greatest challenges to estimating both the shortening fraction and an ejection fraction is the small size of the fetal heart and the reproducibility of measurements. In addition, all measurements require definition of end-diastole and systole, which without an electrocardiogram can be difficult to define.

Diastolic function

Once recognized as the precursor to clinically apparent systolic dysfunction, diastolic dysfunction and its assessment has be at the forefront of fetal imaging today. At present, diastolic performance is assessed by measuring the forward pulsed Doppler tracings of velocities across the mitral valve. Early passive diastolic filling produces the E-wave and active filling during atrial systole produces the A-wave. During fetal life, the majority of diastolic ventricular filling occurs during atrial systole, thus the A-wave is of greater velocity than the E-wave. When diastolic ventricular filling predominantly relies on atrial systole, the magnitude of the A-wave will increase and accordingly, the E/A ratio will decline. A decrease in the E/A ratio and fusion of the two peaks producing a monophasic waveform are considered evidence of decreased cardiac diastolic function. With increasing gestation, the Doppler pattern changes such that by term the tracing mimics that of the postnatal.

Tissue Doppler imaging (TDI) is a relatively new echocardiographic technique that uses traditional Doppler principles to measure the velocity of myocardial motion. Doppler echocardiography relies on the detection of the shift in frequency of ultrasound signals reflected from moving objects. Conventional Doppler assesses the velocity of blood flow by measuring signals from blood cells. In TDI, the same principles are used to quantify myocardial tissue motion.

Global cardiac function

The early recognition of subtle changes in myocardial function is critical. The myocardial performance or Tei index (TI) was introduced in 1995.[22] The TI is calculated from the Doppler waveform obtained by placing the pulsed Doppler sample in the left ventricle at the junction of the anterior leaflet of the mitral valve and the LVOT. It is the sum of the isovolumic contraction time (ICT), defined as the time interval from the end of the A-wave to the onset of the aortic pulsed Doppler tracing, and the isovolumic relaxation time (IRT), defined as the time interval from the end of the aortic pulsed Doppler to the onset of the E-wave, divided by the ejection time (ET), the onset to the end of the aortic pulsed Doppler tracing.

$$TI = (ICT+IRT)/ET$$

The use of the TI in the assessment of fetal function was first reported in 1999 by Tsutsumi and colleagues.[23]

Since its introduction, the utility of the TI in the assessment of global fetal cardiac function has been investigated and normal values have been established.[24] It is an easily obtained, Doppler-derived index that appears to be independent of both gestational age and heart rate.[8,9] It is made up of both systolic (ICT and ET) and diastolic (IRT) components. By incorporating only time intervals, the TI is less dependent on anatomy or precise imaging. There is some variability in reported left ventricular values, with reported normal TI values between 0.35 ± 0.03[25] and 0.53 ± 0.13.[24] If the functional properties of the ventricles decline, an increasing amount of time is spent either building up enough ejection force to open the semilunar valve or relaxing after ejection of blood has been achieved. Either of these developments will produce a shortened ET interval, and longer isovolumetric contraction and relaxation times. Accordingly, an increase in the TI indicates a decrease in global myocardial performance.

APPLICATION OF NEW ULTRASONOGRAPHIC TECHNOLOGY TO FETAL ECHOCARDIOGRAPHY

Cine Loop Capture

Considerable discussion continues as to the utility of cine loop capture rather than solely still frame capture. A comprehensive cardiac evaluation should include sweeps rather than solely a series of still frame captures. Sweeps allow for mental reconstruction and are essential to the understanding of complex cardiac lesions. With the advent of 3-dimensional (3-D) sample volume capture, this may become a moot point in the future.

Three-Dimensional Imaging

Arguably the next ultrasonographic advance to gain widespread acceptance will be 3-D fetal echocardiography. 3-D echocardiography offers potential advantages over conventional 2-D imaging. By acquiring volumetric data sets within a few seconds, 3-D imaging promises to significantly reduce scan time. Compared with 2-D imaging, which may require 30 minutes or more of imaging time in the presence of a complex congenital lesion, 3-D echocardiography with practice may offer a significantly reduced scan-acquisition time of as little as 5 to 10 minutes. 3-D imaging does pose some challenges. The fetus must remain still for 15 to 30 seconds during acquisition and as many as 5 scan sequences may routinely be necessary as part of a complete study. In addition, off-line computer processing remains complicated and time consuming. Finally, fetal 3-D has limitations similar to those encountered with 2-D studies: fetal lie, plane of image acquisition, and late-gestation shadowing from fetal bones and extremities all directly affect the quality of 3-D images.

For screening of low-risk pregnancy, 3-D imaging may allow visualization of the 4-chamber view and outflow tracts from one data set from a single acoustic window. Such a volume data set could then be manipulated, allowing for image plane alignment errors and sonographer inexperience. This potential likely offers the next step in significantly increasing the rate of prenatal diagnosis.

Telemedicine

As expertise in fetal echocardiography may not be available in all communities, unique strategies have been proposed using the rapidly expanding field of telemedicine. Reports of using spatio-temporal image correlation volumes obtained by a nonexpert (general obstetrician) and transmitted electronically via the Internet for remote analysis and interpretation by an expert have emerged.[26–28] As this technology is used more and more, its utility in fetal echocardiography will undoubtedly be realized.

In summary, imaging the fetal heart has evolved significantly since the first reports. Today nearly all women have a screening ultrasound, including cardiac views, during the second trimester and nearly 5% of all women are referred for comprehensive fetal echocardiogram. These detail-oriented examinations can detect and accurately diagnose nearly all forms of congenital heart disease. Serial in utero evaluations combined with postnatal images have provided a natural history of nearly all lesions and have set the stage for fetal intervention, which hopes to alter the observed natural history of the most devastating lesions.

Progress in fetal echocardiography is due in part to gained experience, but also has benefited greatly from technological advances in ultrasonography. In the future, it is likely that 3-D and 4-D fetal echocardiography will further revolutionize the field.

SUPPLEMENTARY DATA

Supplementary data related to this article can be found online at doi:10.1016/j.cult.2011.01.007.

REFERENCES

1. Winsberg F. Echocardiography of the fetal and newborn heart. Invest Radiol 1972;3:152.
2. Sahn DJ, Lange LW, Allen HD, et al. Qualitative real-time cross-sectional echocardiography in the developing human fetus and newborn. Circulation 1980; 62:588.
3. Montana E, Khoury MJ, Cragan JD, et al. Trends and outcomes after prenatal diagnosis of congenital cardiac malformations by fetal echocardiography in a well defined birth population, Atlanta, Georgia, 1990-1994. J Am Coll Cardiol 1996;28:1805–9.
4. Allan LD, Crawford DC, Chita SK, et al. Prenatal screening for congenital heart disease. Br Med J (Clin Res Ed) 1986;292:1717–9.
5. American College of Radiology. ACR practice guidelines for the performance of antepartum obstetrical ultrasound. In Practice Guidelines and Technical Standards. Reston (VA): ACR; 2007.
6. Ultrasonography in Pregnancy. ACOG Practice Bulletin, # 101. Obstet Gynecol 2009;113(2 Pt 1): 451–61.
7. Rychik J, Ayres N, Cuneo B, et al. American Society of Echocardiography guidelines and standards for performance of the fetal echocardiogram. J Am Soc Echocardiogr 2004;17:803–10.
8. Lee W, Drose J, Wax J, et al. AIUM practice guideline for the performance of fetal echocardiography. J Ultrasound Med 2011;30:127–36.
9. Mavrides E, Cobian-Sanchez F, Tekay A, et al. Limitations of using first-trimester nuchal translucency measurement in routine screening for major congenital heart defects. Ultrasound Obstet Gynecol 2001; 17:106–10.
10. Ghi T, Huggon IC, Zosmer N, et al. Incidence of major structural heart defects associated with increased nuchal translucency but normal karyotype. Ultrasound Obstet Gynecol 2001;18:610–4.
11. Smrcek JM, Berg C, Geipel A, et al. Early fetal echocardiography. J Ultrasound Med 2006;25: 173–82.
12. Carvalho JS, Moscoso G, Tekay A, et al. Impact of first and early second trimester fetal echocardiography on high-risk pregnancies. Heart 2004;90:921–6.
13. Trines J, Hornberger LK. Evolution of heart disease in utero. Pediatr Cardiol 2004;25:287–98.
14. Tan J, Silverman NH, Hoffman JI, et al. Cardiac dimensions determined by cross-sectional echocardiography in the normal human fetus from 18 weeks to term. Am J Cardiol 1992;70:1459–67.
15. Sharland GK, Allan LD. Normal fetal cardiac measurements derived by cross-sectional echocardiography. Ultrasound Obstet Gynecol 1992;2: 175–81.
16. Schneider C, McCrindle BW, Carvalho JS, et al. Development of z scores for fetal cardiac dimensions from echocardiography. Ultrasound Obstet Gynecol 2005;26:599–605.
17. Lee W, Riggs T, Amula V, et al. Fetal echocardiography: z-score reference ranges for a large patient population. Ultrasound Obstet Gynecol 2010;35: 28–34.
18. Makikallio K, McElhinney DB, Levine JC, et al. Fetal aortic valve stenosis and the evolution of hypoplastic left heart syndrome: patient selection for fetal intervention. Circulation 2006;113:1401–5.
19. McElhinney DB, Marshall AC, Wilkins-Haug LE, et al. Predictors of technical success and postnatal biventricular outcome after in utero aortic valvuloplasty for aortic stenosis with evolving hypoplastic left heart syndrome. Circulation 2009;120:1482–90.
20. Huhta JC. Guidelines for the evaluation of heart failure in the fetus with or without hydrops. Pediatr Cardiol 2004;25:274–86.
21. Falkensammer CB, Paul J, Huhta JC. Fetal congestive heart failure: correlation of Tei-index and cardiovascular score. J Perinat Med 2001;29:390–8.
22. Tei C, Ling L, Hodge D, et al. New index of combined systolic and diastolic myocardial performance: a simple and reproducible measure of cardiac function—a study in normal and dilated cardiomyopathy. J Cardiol 1995;26:357–66.
23. Tsutsumi T, Ishii M, Eto G, et al. Serial evaluation for myocardial performance in fetuses and neonates using a new Doppler index. Pediatr Int 1999;41:722–7.
24. Friedman D, Buyon J, Kim M, et al. Fetal cardiac function assessed by Doppler myocardial performance index (Tei index). Ultrasound Obstet Gynecol 2003;21:33–6.
25. Eidem BW, Edwards JM, Cetta F. Quantitative assessment of fetal ventricular function: establishing normal values of the myocardial performance index in the fetus. Echocardiography 2001;18:9–13.

26. Viñals F, Mandujano L, Vargas G, et al. Prenatal diagnosis of congenital heart disease using four-dimensional spatiotemporal image correlation (STIC) telemedicine via an Internet link: a pilot study. Ultrasound Obstet Gynecol 2005;25:25–31.

27. Vanals F, Ascenzo R, Naveas R, et al. Fetal Echocardiography at 11 + 0 to 13 + 6 weeks using four-dimensional spatiotemporal image correlation telemedicine via an Internet link: a pilot study. Ultrasound Obstet Gynecol 2008;31:633–8.

28. Michailidis G, Simpson J, Karidas C, et al. Detailed three-dimensional fetal echocardiography facilitated by an Internet link. Ultrasound Obstet Gynecol 2001; 18:325–8.

Fetal Growth Abnormalities

Mariam Moshiri, MD[a],[*], Sophia Rothberger, MD[b]

KEYWORDS

- Twins • Prenatal • Ultrasound

The terminology used to describe abnormal fetal growth in pregnancy is complex and can be confusing. Although defining abnormal fetal growth as the smallest 10% or largest 10% of fetuses for a given gestational age may make statistical sense, this cutoff is not always clinically relevant. In any given population, there is normal variation in size. Thus not all fetuses measuring less than the 10th percentile or greater than the 90th percentile have pathologic growth or adverse outcomes. The most appropriate cutoff for abnormal growth is one that maximizes sensitivity and specificity for adverse perinatal outcomes. Although the specificity for neonatal problems increases with smaller estimated fetal weights (EFWs), using a cutoff of the 10th percentile is more sensitive and more conventionally used.[1]

For further clarity of terminology, a distinction should also be made between abnormal EFW and confirmed birth weight. Although ultrasonographic measurements give a best estimate of the fetal weight in most cases, measurement error does occur and increases with gestational age. Intrauterine growth restriction (IUGR) is a diagnosis made in utero. The term small for gestational age (SGA) is used when the EFW is less than that expected for gestational age but the fetus grows normally. An in utero diagnosis of suspected macrosomia is made when a fetus is estimated to be greater than 4500 g. This diagnosis uses an absolute weight rather than a weight for gestational age because the risk for adverse neonatal outcomes is significant only when an infant's weight is beyond this weight. Large for gestational age (LGA) is considered when the EFW is more than expected for the gestational age but the fetus grows normally.[2,3]

Accurate estimation of the fetal weight has an important role in routine antenatal care as well as detection of fetal growth abnormalities and is therefore an area of significant interest for investigators. Bukowski and colleagues[4] found that the size of the fetus in the first trimester of pregnancy was associated with the birth weight, suggesting that the effect of the first-trimester size on the duration of pregnancy accounted for about half of the association, and fetal growth in later pregnancy accounted for the other half. Pardo and colleagues,[5] in a recent article, suggested a high correlation between crown-rump length (CRL) at 11 to 14 weeks gestation and LGA fetuses (birth weight larger than 90th percentile). They showed that these fetuses are characterized by a larger-than-expected CRL at 11 to 14 weeks gestation by half a week or more. Interestingly, they did not find a smaller-than-expected CRL in pregnancies with SGA neonates.

Most clinicians believe that the major variations in fetal size occur in the second half of pregnancy. Many investigators have suggested various ultrasound-based methods of fetal weight estimation. These methods are based on different combinations of sonographically measured fetal biometric indices: fetal abdominal circumference (AC), biparietal diameter, head circumference, and femur length (FL).[1] Lee and colleagues[6] suggested the use of 3-dimensional ultrasonography to obtain the volumes of one or more fetal body

The author has nothing to disclose.
[a] Division of Radiology, University of Washington Medical Center, University of Washington School of Medicine, 1959 NE Pacific Street, Box 357115, Seattle, WA 98195, USA
[b] Maternal Fetal Medicine, Obstetrics and Gynecology, University of Washington School of Medicine, 1959 NE Pacific Street, Box 357115, Seattle, WA 98195, USA
* Corresponding author.
E-mail address: moshiri@u.washington.edu

Ultrasound Clin 6 (2011) 57–67
doi:10.1016/j.cult.2011.01.008

parts to estimate the fetal weight. Several groups have developed formulas relating these volumes to fetal weight.[7] A recent study by Melamed and colleagues[8] compared many available methods in estimating fetal weight as described in the literature. They found that there is considerable variation among the different sonographic models, although most show good overall accuracy. They also found that for birth weights in the range of 1000 to 4500 g, models based on 3 or 4 fetal biometric indices are better than models that incorporate only 1 or 2 indices. Their results showed that the accuracy of the various models decreases at the extremes of birth weights, resulting in overestimation in low-birth-weight categories and underestimation in birth weights more than 4000 g. They concluded that the precision of the models is lowest in the low-birth-weight groups.

Dudley[9] conducted a review of various methods described in the literature to calculate an EFW. Population differences, maternal factors, and variations in fetal composition were minor issues in the context of the current large random errors in EFW. Image quality is a factor that may be overcome by technological development. Measurement methods and observer variability are major contributors to systemic and random errors. It was suggested that steps in minimizing the variability in EFW can be achieved by standardization of methods, averaging of multiple measurements, improvements in image quality, uniform calibration of equipment, careful design and refinement of measurement methods, and regular audits of measurement quality.[9]

IUGR

IUGR is defined as an EFW less than the 10th percentile. Although it implies impaired fetal growth, the cause cannot be presumed from ultrasonographic measurements alone. IUGR includes normal variability in the size of the population as well as a pathologically small fetus. Both genetic and environmental factors affect fetal growth. IUGR can be fetal, maternal, or primarily placental in origin.[2] **Box 1** lists the clinical conditions associated with a risk of IUGR.

The most common maternal and placental factors inhibit fetal growth by decreasing fetal perfusion either through the microvasculature or through hypoxemia. The maternal conditions include vascular diseases such as hypertension and heart disease, diabetes, drugs, malnutrition, smoking, and alcohol use. Placental factors can compromise fetal growth through a placental genetic component such as confined placental

---

Box 1
Clinical conditions associated with IUGR

Maternal

Uterine abnormalities

Hypertensive and cardiovascular disorders

Renal disease

Hematologic or immunologic disorders

Hypoxemia

Severe malnourishment

Dermatogens or substance exposure

Cigarette smoking

Fetal

Genetic

Chromosomal abnormalities

Congenital anomaly

Multiple gestations

Infection

Placenta

Placental disease

Confined placental mosaics

---

mosaicism, vascular problems such as preeclampsia, or structural problems such as placenta previa or placental abruption. The resulting growth restriction characteristically begins with a small AC and FL, sparing the fetal head. This pattern of growth restriction is termed asymmetric IUGR. However, in severe or chronic circumstances, the fetal head may be affected as well, thus yielding a symmetrically small fetus. Asymmetric IUGR usually presents in the late second to early third trimester of pregnancy.[10,11]

Symmetric IUGR can also occur with intrinsic fetal factors such as genetic predisposition for small size; chromosomal abnormalities such as triploidy and aneuploidy; intrauterine infection with agents such as cytomegalovirus, parvovirus, rubella, and human deficiency virus; and nonaneuploidy syndromes. Symmetric IUGR usually presents in the early second trimester of pregnancy.[12]

Clinical Evaluation

All pregnant women should be screened for fetal growth restriction by fundal height measurements at clinical examinations. These measurements are performed in women after 20 weeks gestation. The sensitivity and specificity of fundal height measurements for detecting IUGR in women without risk factors are similar to those of an

Table 1
IUGR: sample interval growth examination results

	5/12: Baseline Examination (wk/d)	13-wk Interval Expected (wk/d)	8/11 (Actual Examination) (wk/d)	5-wk Interval Expected (wk/d)	9/15 (Actual Examination) (wk/d)
BPD	18/3	31/3	30/3	35/3	35/4
HC	18/2	31/2	31/3	36/3	36/0
AC	18/3	31/3	28/4	33/4	30/4
FL	17/4	30/4	28/4	33/4	33/0
—	—	—	Fetal weight, 23%	—	Fetal weight <10%

Abbreviations: BPD, biparietal diameter; FL, femur length; HC, head circumference.

obstetric ultrasonography. However, women with a previous SGA infant or other significant risk factors for delivering an SGA infant should undergo an obstetric ultrasonography to evaluate fetal growth. Although generally ultrasound examinations are performed early in the third trimester, the frequency and timing of these examinations have not been clearly established. The sensitivity for detecting IUGR can be improved by the use of serial ultrasound examinations to evaluate the trajectory of growth.[13,14]

Ultrasound Evaluation

Determining an accurate gestational age before assessment for IUGR is important because it can be used as a reference while measuring fetal biometric indices. If a first-trimester examination is available, then the estimated gestational age on that examination can be used as the reference. Otherwise, the gestational age based on the last menstrual period can be used. Fetal biometric indices should be measured to calculate an estimated gestational age. These parameters can then be used on interval follow-up examinations to determine whether the fetus has grown appropriately in the interval. Serial biometry is the recommended gold standard for assessing pregnancies at a high risk for IUGR (**Table 1**).[13]

In fetuses with early IUGR, there is redistribution of the intrahepatic venous flow, with shunting of blood flow away from the right lobe of the liver. This shunting is associated with decreased glycogen storage in the liver and a decrease in the size of the fetal AC, the first ultrasonographic sign of IUGR. This sign appears before the composite EFW reduces to less than the 10th percentile (**Table 2**).[10] Changes in the fetal circulation also result in decreased renal perfusion and therefore decreased fetal urine production. Therefore, IUGR is also associated with oligohydramnios.[15,16]

Table 2
Early IUGR: the fetal AC measurement is below the accepted standard deviation for EGA, but the fetal weight is not less than 10%

Fetal Biometry	Baseline Examination: 7/18 (cm)	Growth Parameters (wk/d)	Follow-up Examination: 8/8 Expected Growth in 3-Wk Interval (wk/d)	Actual Examination (cm)	Actual Growth Parameters (wk/d)
BPD	6.5	26/1	29/1	7.5	29/4
HC	24.2	26/2	29/1	26.7	28/1
AC	16.6	21/4	24/4	28.9	25/2
FL	4.1	23/3	26/3	5.1	27/0
—	EFW: 685 g for EGA of 26/2 by LMP	EFW: 15%	—	EFW: 1015 g for EGA of 29/2 by LMP	EFW: <10%

Abbreviations: BPD, biparietal diameter; EFW, estimated fetal weight; EGA, estimated gestational age; FL, femur length; HC, head circumference; LMP, last menstrual period.

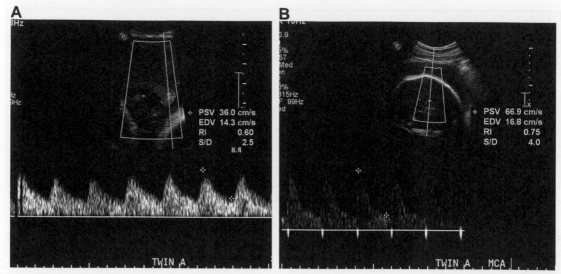

Fig. 1. Normal fetal Doppler. (*A*) Normal low-resistance flow in the uterine artery. (*B*) Normal middle cerebral artery (MCA) Doppler. Normal high-resistance flow in the MCA. The ratio of MCA S/D to that of umbilical artery S/D is normal and greater than 1.5 in this patient. EDV, end diastolic velocity; PSV, peak systolic velocity; RI: resistive index.

An elevation in placental blood flow resistance and a decrease in blood flow resistance in the cerebral circulation produce a decrease in the cerebroplacental Doppler ratio. These changes can be measured by determining the systolic/diastolic (S/D) ratio of the Doppler waveforms for the umbilical artery and middle cerebral artery (MCA) (**Fig. 1**). The relative ratio of the MCA to uterine artery (UA) S/D parameter should remain more than 1.5 in normal fetal circulatory conditions (**Figs. 2** and **3**). With progressive placental villous obliteration, the placental blood flow resistance progressively increases. When villous obliteration affects more than half the placenta, umbilical artery end-diastolic flow may be absent or reversed. These changes result in significant fetal central circulatory effects with resultant preference for fetal myocardium and cerebral circulation (**Figs. 4** and **5**).[10,17]

During early IUGR, no flow changes are seen in the fetal cerebral circulation. However, with increased resistance of flow in the placenta, the flow resistance in the cerebral circulation decreases. This effect can be demonstrated on Doppler examination of the MCA. With progressive IUGR and placental villous obliteration, there is an increased preference for cerebral circulation and a resultant low resistance flow, the so-called

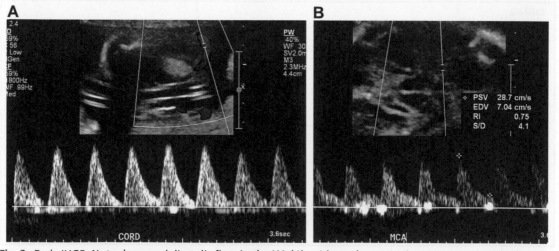

Fig. 2. Early IUGR. Note decreased diastolic flow in the UA (*A*), with no change in the MCA Doppler (*B*). The ratio of MCA S/D to umbilical artery S/D is greater than 1.5.

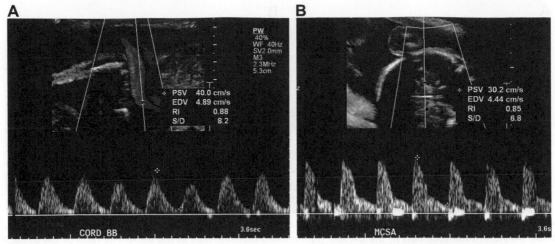

Fig. 3. Advanced IUGR. The ratio of MCA S/D to umbilical artery S/D is now less than 1.5 at 0.8 (*A, B*).

head sparing.[10,11,18] In advanced IUGR, there is an increased fetal ventricular after-load, which can eventually result in cardiac decompensation. Once reversed end-diastolic flow is seen in the umbilical artery, progression to late manifestations of central venous flow patterns can be observed. These include reversal of flow in the fetal *inferior vena cava*, reversal of *a* wave in ductus venosus, and pulsatile flow in the umbilical vein (**Fig. 6**).[10,11,19]

In early IUGR, fetal development in a chronic state of relative nutrition and oxygen deprivation produces a measurable delay in the achievement of behavioral milestones. These include relative increase in fetal baseline heart rate, lower heart rate variability and variation, and delayed achievement of heart rate reactivity. In late IUGR, biophysical parameters become abnormal in a sequential manner, which is determined by the relative sensitivity of the central regulatory centers to a decline

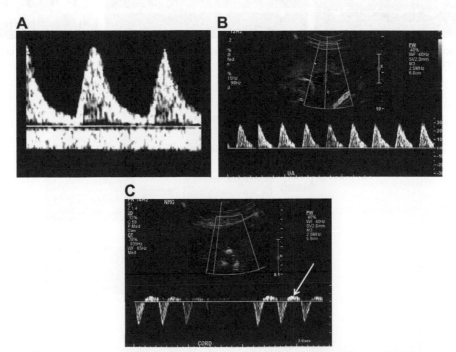

Fig. 4. Fetal UA Doppler. With elevated resistance in the placenta, there is progression of high-resistance flow in the UA. (*A*) Decreased diastolic flow. (*B*) Absent diastolic flow. (*C*) Reversal of diastolic flow (arrow points to the reversal component).

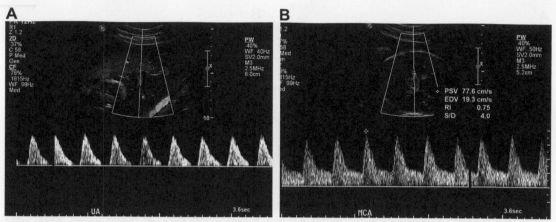

Fig. 5. Effects of placental insufficiency on UA and MCA Doppler with resultant lowered resistance flow in the MCA. (*A*) Absent diastolic flow in the UA and (*B*) increased diastolic flow in the MCA. The ratio of UA to MCA S/D parameter is less than 1.5.

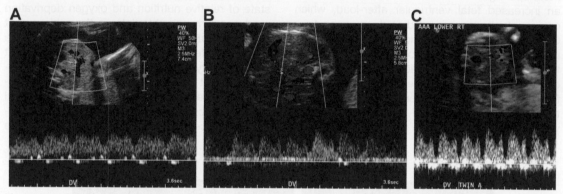

Fig. 6. Doppler of ductus venosus. (*A*) Normal flow. (*B*) Increased impedance to flow. (*C*) Absent end-diastolic flow with transient partial reversal.

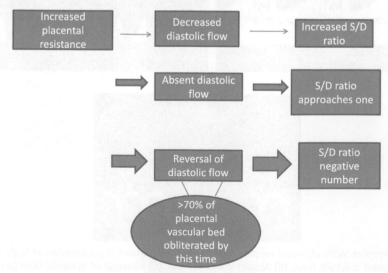

Fig. 7. Fetal UA Doppler trends in progressive IUGR.

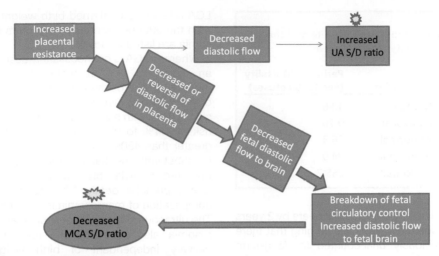

Fig. 8. Fetal MCA and umbilical artery Doppler.

in fetal pH.[20] Accordingly, loss of fetal heart rate reactivity precedes loss of breathing, gross body movement, and tone.[10] Such changes in the fetus can be assessed by ultrasound examination as well.

Fetal nonstress test (NST) is usually performed after 28 weeks of gestation. This test is used to evaluate fetal cardiac response to its own movements and reflects adequate blood flow and proper oxygenation of the fetus. A nonreactive NST points to fetal distress. Other abnormalities on NST suggesting fetal distress include fetal cardiac decelerations, fetal tachycardia, and absence of reactivity (**Figs. 7** and **8**).[21]

The fetal biophysical profile monitors fetal response to the environment. Four parameters are measured, each carrying a maximum score of 2: fetal breathing, fetal movement, cardiac reactivity, and volume of amniotic fluid. In general, acute fetal hypoxia as can be seen in early IUGR is commonly associated with abnormalities of

movement and tone (**Tables 3** and **4**).[22–24] Blood flow velocity does not change in fetuses with fetal factor IUGR such as chromosomal abnormalities and is therefore not useful in these circumstances.

Perinatal Morbidity and Mortality

Neonates born with SGA have an increased risk of morbidity and mortality. Studies have shown that the mortality rate in term infants increases as the weight for gestational age decreases, with a clear difference in perinatal mortality by the third percentile. There is also an increased risk for respiratory distress and sepsis in these infants. Morbidity and mortality for preterm infants born SGA is higher than for term infants.[25,26] Long-term effects are associated with the cause of low birth weight. For example, genetic abnormalities or congenital infection is more predictive of neonatal outcomes than the infant's birth weight. Most SGA infants without other comorbidities are

Table 3
Components of a 30-min biophysical profile

Component	Definition
Fetal movements	≥3 body or limb movements
Fetal tone	1 episode of active extension and flexion of the limbs; opening and closing of hand
Fetal breathing movement	≥1 episode of ≥30 s in 30 min; hiccups are considered breathing activity
AFI	A single 2 × 2-cm pocket is considered adequate
Each get a score of 2	Total score of 8
NST	2 accelerations >15 beats per minute of at least 15-s duration.

Abbreviations: AFI, amniotic fluid index; NST, nonstress test.

Table 4
Distribution of biophysical profile and the perinatal mortality associated with it

Score	Description	Perinatal Mortality (Per 1000 Fetuses)
8–10	Normal	1.86
6	Equivocal	9.76
4	Abnormal	26.3
2	Abnormal	94.0
0	Abnormal	255.7

able to catch up in weight to their peers by 2 years of age, but some evidence is emerging that there may be previously unaccounted for long-term sequelae. Studies suggest an increased risk for hypertension and cardiovascular disease, cerebral palsy, and other adverse neurologic outcomes in low-birth-weight infants.[27–30]

Adjunct ultrasonographic parameters can be useful in further determining fetal risk of stillbirth. The presence of oligohydramnios in the setting of IUGR increases the risk of fetal death. However, the absence of oligohydramnios does not preclude fetal and neonatal risk.[31] Intervention guided by abnormal umbilical arterial velocimetry in conjunction with other antenatal testing has been shown to reduce perinatal deaths. Specifically, the absence or reversal of end-diastolic flow is associated with increased perinatal morbidity and mortality as well as long-term neurologic outcomes. In contrast, those fetuses with normal values in Doppler velocimetry do not appear to exhibit those adverse outcomes, and unnecessary intervention can be avoided with normal findings.

Once IUGR is detected, growth should be followed serially in conjunction with additional antenatal testing to determine optimal delivery timing. No antenatal interventions aside from optimizing delivery timing have been shown to reduce neonatal morbidity and mortality. These follow-up ultrasound examinations are most useful when separated by enough time to reduce ultrasound measurement error (typically intervals of 2–4 weeks). Serial ultrasound examinations should be performed in conjunction with antenatal testing such as amniotic fluid index, biophysical profile, fetal heart rate monitoring, and Doppler velocimetry.[32,33]

FETAL MACROSOMIA

Fetal macrosomia is a diagnosis made in pregnancy to describe an EFW of greater than 4000 or 4500 g, depending on the threshold used.

LGA refers to a confirmed birth weight of greater than the 90th percentile.[3] Risk factors for macrosomia are listed in **Box 2**.

Whereas LGA is not necessarily associated with an increased risk of maternal and neonatal morbidity, macrosomia is. The risk of shoulder dystocia and resulting neonatal injuries increases significantly with macrosomia, from a low baseline risk of 1.4% to 9%–24% with a birth weight of greater than 4500 g. Shoulder dystocia can lead to substantial neonatal complications including fractured clavicle, brachial plexus injury, and, rarely, prenatal death.[34–36] The most frequent complication of macrosomia is cesarean delivery. The ultrasound diagnosis of suspected fetal macrosomia also increases the risk of cesarean delivery independent of birth weight. Other maternal risks associated with macrosomia include vaginal lacerations and postpartum hemorrhage. Unfortunately, interventions for suspected fetal macrosomia have not successfully reduced adverse outcomes. Several studies have shown that performing a cesarean section for suspected macrosomia significantly increases the cesarean rate without eliminating the risk of shoulder dystocia injuries. However, the American Congress of Obstetrics and Gynecology does recommend that practitioners consider prophylactic cesarean delivery in patients with suspected fetal weight of greater than 5000 g or greater than 4500 g when the patient has diabetes. One study showed that it would take 2345 cesarean deliveries to prevent 1 permanent injury. Induction of labor for anticipated macrosomia also does not reduce the risk of shoulder dystocia or birth injury and may actually increase the risk of cesarean delivery.[37–41]

In women with risk factors or suspected macrosomia by clinical examination, an ultrasound examination can be performed to estimate fetal weight. On ultrasound examination, fetal biometry is used to estimate the fetal weight (**Table 5**). In macrosomic fetuses, increased subcutaneous fat is observed, which appears as echogenic tissue (**Fig. 9**). Truncal obesity is also commonly

Box 2
Risk factors for macrosomia

Prior history of macrosomia

Diabetes

Maternal obesity

Maternal weight gain

Gestational age greater than 40 weeks

Table 5
Fetal macrosomia: sample growth measurements in a fetus with macrosomia

	Baseline Examination: 7/18 (cm)	Growth Parameters (wk/d)	Follow-up Examination: 8/8 Expected Growth Parameters in the 3-wk Interval (wk/d)	Actual Examination (cm)	Actual Examination: Estimated Growth (wk/d)
BPD	6.9	27/4	30/4	7.9	31/4
HC	25.2	27/2	30/2	28.1	29/5
AC	22.6	27/0	30/0	28	31/5
FL	5	27/0	30/0	6.2	32/0
—	EFW: 1039 g for EGA 26/2	Fetal EFW is within 75%	—	EFW: 1892 g for EGA 29/2 based on LMP	Fetal EFW is >90%

Abbreviations: BPD, biparietal diameter; EGA, estimated gestational age; FL, femur length; HC, head circumference; LMP, last menstrual period.

observed. Unfortunately, ultrasound measurement error increases with gestational age and fetal weight, with the error exceeding 10%. In addition, maternal obesity, a common risk factor for macrosomia, further increases ultrasound error, making for a diagnostic challenge in a high-risk population.

For these reasons, optimal timing for the ultrasound examination is not clear.[42–44]

In conclusion, accurate assessment of EFW can be compromised by several factors including operator and observer variabilities. Measures should be taken to minimize these variables.

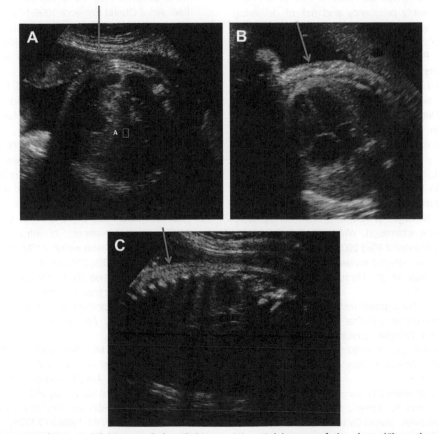

Fig. 9. Macrosomic fetus. Axial image of the abdomen (*A*), axial image of the chest (*B*), and coronal image through the chest (*C*). Note the subcutaneous echogenic fat (*arrow*).

Once IUGR is suspected, there are several ultrasound-based examinations that can assist clinicians in the management of the pregnancy. Because the best current treatment for IUGR is delivery of the fetus, all diagnostic measures should be used to optimize the decision on the timing of the delivery. Fetal macrosomia is associated with perinatal morbidity both for the fetus and the mother. Ultrasound examination is helpful for the assessment of fetal macrosomia but not conclusive. Further investigation for a more definitive diagnostic method is needed.

REFERENCES

1. Benacerraf BR, Gelman R, Frigoletto FD Jr. Sonographically estimated fetal weights: accuracy and limitation. Am J Obstet Gynecol 1988;159:1118.
2. American College of Obstetrics and Gynecology: intrauterine growth restriction. ACOG Practice Bulletin No 12. Washington, DC: American College of Obstetrics and Gynecology; 2000.
3. Fetal macrosomia. Number 22. ACOG Practice Bulletin 2000. Reaffirmed 2010.
4. Bukowski R, Smith GC, Malone FD, et al. Fetal growth in early pregnancy and risk of delivering low birth weight infant: prospective cohort study. BMJ 2007;334:836–9.
5. Pardo J, Peled Y, Yogev Y, et al. Association of crown-rump length at 11 to 14 weeks' gestation and risk of a large-for-gestational-age neoate. J Ultrasound Med 2010;29:1315–9.
6. Lee W, Deter RL, Ebersole JD, et al. Birth weight prediction by three-dimensional ultrasonography: fractional limb volume. J Ultrasound Med 2001;20: 1283–92.
7. Schild RL, Fimmers R, Hansmann M. Fetal weight estimation by three-dimensional ultrasound. Ultrasound Obstet Gynecol 2000;16:445–52.
8. Melamed N, Yogev Y, Meizner I, et al. Sonographic fetal weight estimation. Which model should be used? J Ultrasound Med 2009;28:617–29.
9. Dudley NJ. A systemic review of the ultrasound estimation of fetal weight. Ultrasound Obstet Gynecol 2005;25:80–9.
10. Baschat AA. Fetal growth restriction—from observation to intervention. J Perinat Med 2010;38:239–46.
11. Baschat AA. Doppler application in delivery timing of the preterm growth-restricted fetus: another step in the right direction. Ultrasound Obstet Gynecol 2004;23:111–8.
12. Dashe JS, McIntire DD, Lucas MJ, et al. Effects of symmetric and asymmetric fetal growth on pregnancy outcomes. Obstet Gynecol 2000;96(3):321–7.
13. Figueras F, Gardosi J. Intrauterine growth restriction: new concepts in antenatal surveillance, diagnosis, and management. Am J Obstet Gynecol 2011. [Epub ahead of print].
14. Chauhan SP, Hendrix NW, Magann EF, et al. Limitations of clinical and sonographic estimates of birth weight: experience with 1034 parturients. Obstet Gynecol 1998;91:72.
15. Varma TR, Bateman S, Patel RH, et al. Ultrasound evaluation of amniotic fluid: outcome of pregnancies with severe oligohydramnios. Int J Gynaecol Obstet 1988;27:185.
16. Philipson EH, Sokol RJ, Williams T. Oligohydramnios: clinical associations and predictive value for intrauterine growth retardation. Am J Obstet Gynecol 1983;146:271.
17. Davies JA, Gallivan S, Spencer JA. Randomised controlled trial of Doppler ultrasound screening of placental perfusion during pregnancy. Lancet 1992;340:1299.
18. Karsdorp VH, van Vugt JM, van Geijn HP, et al. Clinical significance of absent or reversed end-diastolic velocity waveforms in the umbilical artery. Lancet 1994;334:1664.
19. Krebs C, Marca LM, Leiser RL, et al. Intrauterine growth restriction with absent end-diastolic flow velocity in the umbilical artery is associated with maldevelopment of the placental terminal villous tree. Am J Obstet Gynecol 1996;175:1534.
20. Nicolaides KH, Bilardp CM, Soothill PW, et al. Absence of end-diastolic frequencies in umbilical artery: a sign of fetal hypoxia and acidosis. BMJ 1988;297:1026.
21. Cosmi E, Berghella V, Funai E, et al. Doppler, NST, and biophysical profile changes in idiopathic IUGR fetuses—a longitudinal multicenter study. Am J Obstet Gynecol 2005;193(6):S133.
22. Ott WJ, Mora G, Arias F, et al. Comparison of the modified biophysical profile to a "new" biophysical profile incorporating the middle cerebral artery to umbilical artery velocity flow systolic diastolic ratio. Am J Obstet Gynecol 1998;178:1346.
23. Kaur S, Picconi JL, Chadha R, et al. Biophysical profile in the treatment of intrauterine growth-restricted fetuses who weigh <1000g. Am J Obstet Gynecol 2008;199(3):264, e1–4.
24. Odibo AO, Quinones JN, Lawrence-Cleary K, et al. What antepartum fetal test should guide the timing of delivery of the preterm growth-restricted fetus? A decision-analysis. Am J Obstet Gynecol 2004; 191(4):1477–82.
25. Craigo SD, Beach ML, Harvey-Wilkes KB, et al. Ultrasound predictors of neonatal outcome in intrauterine growth restriction. Am J Perinatol 1996;13:465.
26. McIntire DD, Bloom SL, Casey BM, et al. Birth weight in relation to morbidity and mortality among newborn infants. N Engl J Med 1999;340:1234.
27. Hadders-Algra M, Towen BC. Body measurements, neurologic and behavioral development in six year

old children born preterm and/or small-for-gestational age. Early Hum Dev 1990;22:1.

28. Low JA, Handley-Derry MH, Burke SO, et al. Association of intrauterine fetal growth retardation and learning deficits at age 9 to 11 years. Am J Obstet Gynecol 1992;167:1499.

29. Smelder C, Faxelius G, Bremme K, et al. Psychological development in children born with very low birth weight after severe intrauterine growth retardation: a 10-year follow-up study. Acta Paediatr 1992;81:197.

30. Barker DJ, Osmond C, Golding J, et al. Growth in utero, blood pressure in childhood and adult life, and mortality from cardiovascular diseases. BMJ 1989;298:564.

31. Chamberlain PF, Manning FA, Morrison I, et al. Ultrasound evaluation of amniotic fluid volume. I. The relationship of marginal and decreased amniotic fluid on perinatal outcome. Am J Obstet Gynecol 1984;150:245.

32. Pattison RC, Norman K, Odendal HJ. The role of Doppler velocimetry in the management of high-risk pregnancies. Br J Obstet Gynaecol 1994;101:114.

33. Omtzigt AM, Reuwer PJ, Bruinse HW. A randomized controlled trial on the clinical value of umbilical Doppler velocimetry in antenatal care. Am J Obstet Gynecol 1994;170:625.

34. Bérard J, Dufour P, Vinatier D, et al. Fetal macrosomia: risk factors and outcome. A study of the outcome concerning 100 cases >4500 g. Eur J Obstet Gynecol Reprod Biol 1998;77:51.

35. Shoulder dystocia. Number 40. ACOG Practice Bulletin 2002. Reaffirmed 2010.

36. Nocon JJ, McKenzie DK, Thomas LJ, et al. Shoulder dystocia: an analysis of risks and obstetric maneuvers. Am J Obstet Gynecol 1993;168:1732.

37. Stones RW, Paterson CM, Saunders NJ. Risk factors for major obstetric haemorrhage. Eur J Obstet Gynecol Reprod Biol 1993;48:15.

38. Leaphart WL, Meyer MC, Capeless EL. Labor induction with a prenatal diagnosis of fetal macrosomia. J Matern Fetal Med 1997;6:99.

39. Gonen O, Rosen DJ, Dolfin Z, et al. Induction of labor versus expectant management in macrosomia: a randomized study. Obstet Gynecol 1997;89:913.

40. Delpapa EH, Mueller-Heubach E. Pregnancy outcome following ultrasound diagnosis of macrosomia. Obstet Gynecol 1991;78:340.

41. Rouse DJ, Owen J, Goldenberg RL, et al. The effectiveness and costs of elective cesarean delivery for fetal macrosomia diagnosed by ultrasound. JAMA 1996;276:1480.

42. Deter RL, Hadlock FP. Use of ultrasound in the detection of macrosomia: a review. J Clin Ultrasound 1985;13:519.

43. Levine AB, Lockwood CJ, Brown B, et al. Sonographic diagnosis of the large for gestational age fetus at term: does it make a difference? Obstet Gynecol 1992;79:55.

44. Johnstone FD, Prescott RJ, Steel JM, et al. Clinical and ultrasound prediction of macrosomia in diabetic pregnancy. Br J Obstet Gynaecol 1996;103:747.

Fetal MR Imaging

Manjiri Dighe, MD

KEYWORDS

- Fetal • MR imaging • Magnetic resonance imaging
- Prenatal

Ultrasonography is the first technique used for fetal imaging because of its proven utility, widespread availability, and relatively low cost. However, ultrasonography has limitations that include a small field of view, limited soft-tissue acoustic contrast, beam attenuation by adipose tissue, poor image quality in oligohydramnios, and limited visualization of the intracranial structures after 33 weeks' gestation because of calvarial calcification. Magnetic resonance (MR) imaging during pregnancy was first described in 1983 with mainly maternal and placental applications.[1] MR imaging is increasingly and frequently used for the prenatal evaluation of fetuses, due to the development of the single-shot rapid acquisition sequence with refocused echoes. MR imaging technology has improved significantly over the past several years, becoming much faster, hence decreasing scan time and increasing image quality. With the introduction of faster sequences, the need for sedation has almost been eliminated, and consistent and high-quality images can now be obtained. MR imaging, however, has to be used as an adjunct to ultrasonography. A study by Santos and colleagues[2] found that in cases where MR imaging was performed after an ultrasonogram, in 42.7% findings on MR imaging were concordant with the referral diagnosis, in 29.3% of cases MR imaging completely changed the diagnosis, and in 28% additional findings were seen. In addition to MR imaging being used for diagnosis, it is also used increasingly for prenatal assessment for fetal or immediate postnatal surgery. This article outlines the various techniques and applications of MR imaging in fetal imaging.

SAFETY OF FETAL MR IMAGING

Concerns of safety of MR imaging arise for both the fetus and mother. Maternal safety concerns are the same as for a nonpregnant patient, and are addressed by standard MR imaging screening. Fetal safety concerns are related to teratogenesis and acoustic damage. MR imaging can be safely performed in pregnancy. Surveys of children exposed to MR imaging in utero[3] and those born to pregnant MR imaging workers found no adverse fetal outcome.[4] The guidelines of the National Radiological Protection Board in the United Kingdom[5] state that "it might be prudent to exclude pregnant women during the first 3 months of pregnancy." The Safety Committee of the Society of Magnetic Resonance Imaging concluded that prenatal MR imaging is indicated when other nonionizing diagnostic imaging methods are inadequate or when the MR examination provides important information that would otherwise require the use of ionizing radiation.[6] Loud noises can be generated by the coils of an MR scanner, which can potentially cause acoustic damage to the fetus. Two reports from United Kingdom provide reassuring clinical and experimental evidence that the risk of acoustic injury is negligible.[3,7] Because gadolinium chelates have been shown to cross the placenta, they are not advised to be used during pregnancy. Gadolinium chelates appear in the fetal bladder and are thus reabsorbed from the amniotic fluid by swallowing, leading to recirculation. Therefore the biologic half-life of gadolinium in the fetus is not known.[6] Consent is routinely obtained, and patients are informed of the lack of conclusive proof regarding safety of fetal MR imaging.

TECHNIQUE

Fetal MR imaging should be performed on 1.5-T MR imaging scanner using a large surface phased array coil. Safety of higher field strengths for this application has not been proven and should

Financial disclosures: None.
Department of Radiology, University of Washington, 1959 NE Pacific Street, Box 357115, Seattle, WA 98195, USA
E-mail address: dighe@u.washington.edu

Ultrasound Clin 6 (2011) 69–85
doi:10.1016/j.cult.2011.01.001

preferably be avoided. Fasting for 4 hours can help reduce bowel peristalsis artifacts and prevent postprandial fetal motion. Voiding immediately before the examination helps avoid discomfort from a full bladder. To avoid compression on the vena cava and its consequences, especially in the latter half of gestation, the pregnant patient should usually be placed in a left lateral decubitus position.

The fetal MR examination should be started with a localizer in 3 planes, preferably with a T2-weighted sequence because it provides more information about the fetus than T1-weighted images. The authors acquire a 3-plane Balanced fast field echo (FFE) sequence (scan time 18

seconds) to obtain an orientation of the fetal lie (**Fig. 1**). Fetuses may not restrict themselves to the exact anatomic planes within the mother, and localization is important to then acquire anatomically correct images of the fetus. It is important to remember that in fetal MR imaging all subsequent scans need to be oriented to the fetal axes and not the maternal axes. The mainstay of fetal MR imaging is generally single-shot T2-weighted sequences such as a true fast imaging steady precession or balanced gradient echo (BFFE), or a half-Fourier acquired single-shot turbo spin-echo (HASTE) sequence. In general, the specific absorption rate (SAR) is significantly lower with fast imaging with steady-state free procession

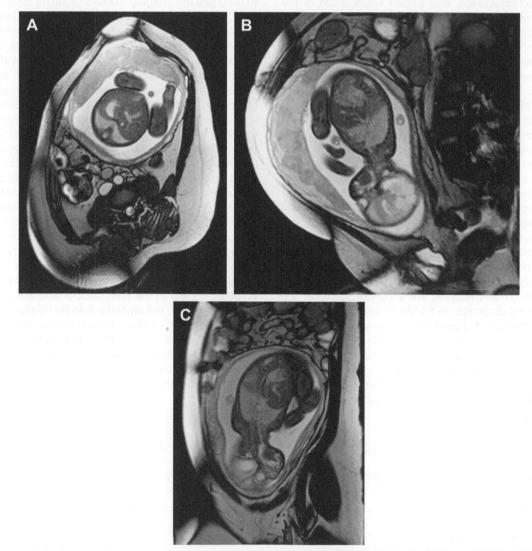

Fig. 1. Multiplanar balanced FFE images (A, axial, B, sagittal; C, coronal) acquired used for planning the dedicated images on the fetus.

Table 1
Typical protocol used at the University of Washington Medical Center for fetal MR imaging

Survey sequence	B-FFE	TE: 1.84 shortest TR: 3.7 shortest FA: 60 ST: 7.0 mm NSA: 1	Matrix: 234/256 Minimum FOV: 400
Sense scan		Used in single-shot sequences with long acquisition	
T2 SSH TSE	Axial, coronal, and sagittal Axial—perpendicular to midbrain Sagittal—parallel to midbrain	TE: 100 TR: 7550 FA: 90 ST: 4.0/0.4 mm NSA: 1	Matrix: 256/256 Minimum FOV: 325
T1 2D GRE	Axial	TE: 3.8 TR: 7.7 FA: 21 ST: 5.0/0.5 mm	Matrix: 199/256 Minimum FOV: 300 NSA: 1–3

Abbreviations: B-FFE, balanced fast field echo; FA, flip angle; FOV, field of view; GRE, gradient echo imaging; NSA, number of signal averages; SSH, single-shot; ST, slice thickness; TE, echo time; TR, repetition time; TSE, turbo spin echo.

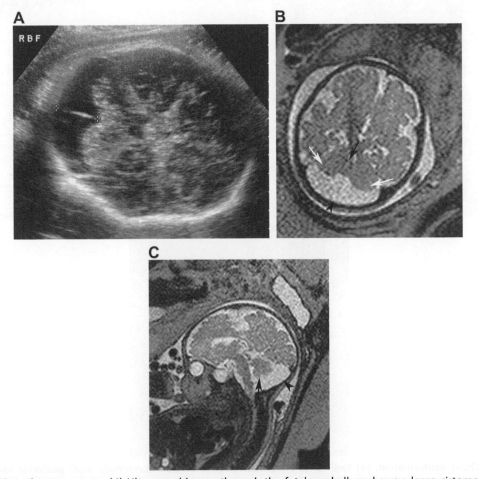

Fig. 2. Megacisterna magna. (*A*) Ultrasound image through the fetal cerebellum shows a large cisterna magna (calipers) measuring 2.3 cm in size. (*B*) Axial and (*C*) sagittal T2-weighted images from a fetal MR image through the posterior fossa show a normal cerebellum (*arrow*) and vermis (*black arrow*) with a large posterior fossa cyst (*black arrowhead*). This was a megacisterna magna. The rest of the intracranial anatomy was normal.

(true FISP) as compared with HASTE sequences under equivalent imaging conditions.[8] The sequences should be performed in the region of interest in all 3 planes. Even though the image quality is significantly lower than the single-shot T2-weighted sequences, a T1-weighted sequence should also be performed to look for hemorrhage. Different types of T1-weighted sequences are available for use in fetal MR imaging. At present, fast low-angle shot (FLASH) sequences are the most robust and commonly used ones. The newest generation of MR scanners now allow the acquisition of 3-dimensional (3D), T2-weighted, single-shot sequences such as a 3D true-FISP sequence. The advantage of 3D acquisition is the speed with which the scanners can acquire the data and hence considerably reduce the examination time to less than

10 minutes, and their multiplanar capability. Without the 3D single-shot sequences, a routine fetal MR examination with a detailed depiction of both the region of interest and the whole body in 3 planes takes less than 20 to 25 minutes. A typical scan protocol used at the author's institution is outlined in **Table 1**. Additional sequences such as diffusion-weighted imaging, echoplanar imaging (EPI), fluid-attenuated inversion recovery (FLAIR) sequences, and dynamic cine sequences can also be used.[9]

INDICATIONS

MR imaging has been used to evaluate almost all the fetal anatomy with the exception of the fetal heart, which is too small for adequate resolution. Major indications for fetal MR imaging include

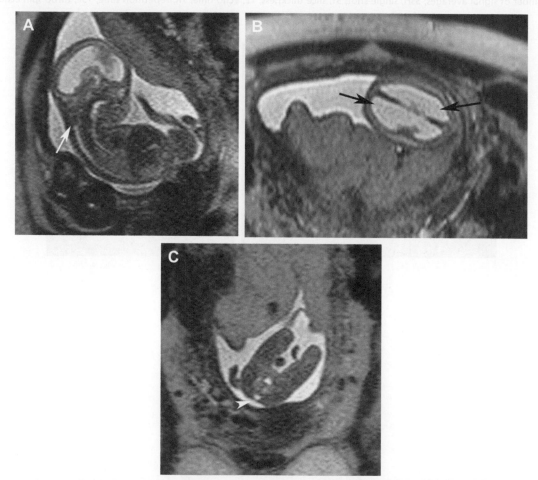

Fig. 3. Chiari malformation. (A) Sagittal T2-weighted image shows an abnormally small posterior fossa with crowding of the cerebellum with effacement of the craniocervical junction (*arrow*). (B) Axial T2-weighted image shows severe bilateral hydrocephalus (*black arrows*). (C) Axial image through the lower lumbar spine shows a small bony defect (*arrowhead*) with a very small cystic structure dorsal to the skin consistent with a small myelomeningocele (not shown).

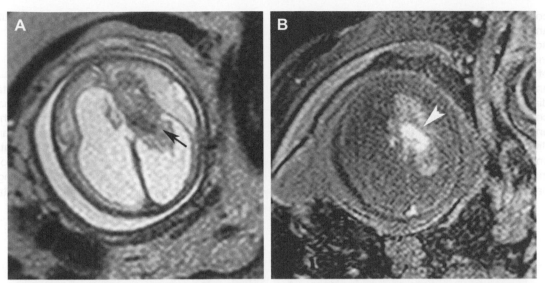

Fig. 4. Intracranial hemorrhage. Fetus with asymmetric ventriculomegaly found on follow up studies. (*A*) Axial T2-weighted fetal MR image shows dilatation of the both ventricles with mild thinning of the overlying cortex and heterogeneous areas in the left ventricle (*arrow*). (*B*) T1-weighted image shows increased signal intensity within this ventricle suggesting hemorrhage (*arrowhead*).

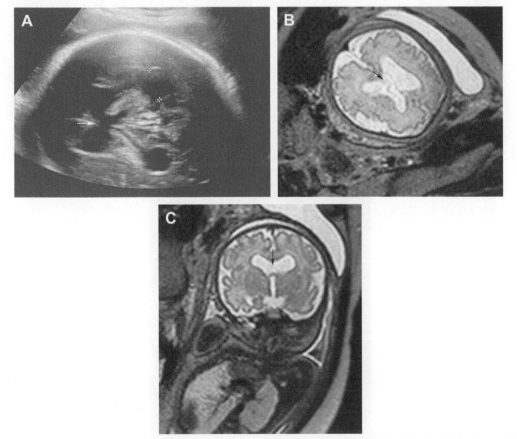

Fig. 5. Absent cavum septum pellucidum. (*A*) Ultrasound image through the fetal head demonstrates absent septum pellucidum (*arrow*) with mild ventriculomegaly (calipers). Axial (*B*) and coronal (*C*) T2-weighted images from fetal MR imaging through the brain in a fetus with absent cavum septum pellucidum (*arrow*). The rest of the intracranial anatomy was normal.

confirmation of inconclusive ultrasound findings and evaluation of sonographically occult diagnosis. In the study by Santos and colleagues,[2] most frequent indications included abnormalities of the central nervous system (CNS) (38%) and lung/thoracic cavity (34%), with congenital diaphragmatic hernia (CDH) the single most common referral diagnosis (17%). Normal fetal anatomy, especially of the fetal brain, is quite different from that seen on ultrasonography, and knowledge of the same is necessary to avoid mistakes in interpretation of normal findings as pathology. Normal fetal anatomy and some of

the pathology seen on fetal MR imaging is outlined in this section.

Central Nervous System and Spine

Ultrasonography is limited in evaluating the fetal brain because of the overlying calvarium that hampers visualization of the brain close to the transducer, technical factors, nonspecific appearance of some anomalies, and lack of adequate differentiation of the gray and white matter on ultrasonography as compared with MR imaging. Reasons for performing MR imaging of the fetal

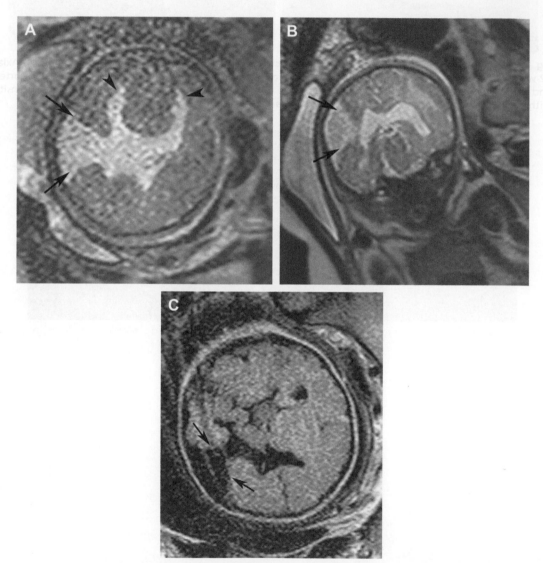

Fig. 6. Schizencephaly. Axial (A) and coronal (B) T2-weighted images, and axial T1-weighted image (C) show a defect along the right cerebral hemisphere (*arrow*) which is either a schizencephaly or porencephalic cyst. Fetus also had an absent cavum septum pellucidum. Notice the colpocephaly (*arrowhead*). Postnatal MR imaging showed this to be an absent septum pellucidum with schizencephaly.

brain include improved assessment of many intracranial structures by MR imaging as compared with ultrasonography, lack of artifacts from overlying ossified skull, and increased familiarity of surgeons who are involved in counseling of parents and treatment of these fetuses/babies with MR imaging as compared with ultrasonography. A study that compared subsequent MR imaging in 124 fetuses with CNS anomalies showed changes in counseling and diagnosis and clear changes in management in 73, 46, and 27 cases, respectively.[10] Another study in which MR imaging was performed when CNS anomalies were suspected on ultrasonography found additional findings in 64%, altered diagnosis in 28%, and changes in management in 11%.[11]

When evaluating fetal brain, it is important to remember that the fetal brain structures are not developed completely and that the imaging appearance will depend on the gestational age at which the fetus is imaged. Fetal gyration does not start until 22 weeks, and the fetal brain appears "smooth" before this gestational age.[12] The fetal brain is also not myelinated, and myelination does not complete until approximately 10 to 12 months of postnatal age. Hence the signal intensity of the fetal white matter is hyperintense on T2-weighted sequences and should not be mistaken for pathologic features such as leukoencephalopathy. Subarachnoid spaces can remain large throughout pregnancy, particularly in the posterior parieto-occipital regions, because of the evolving process of cavitation of the meninx primitiva.[13]

MR imaging is more reliable in detecting the cause of ventriculomegaly and other abnormalities associated with ventriculomegaly,[14] in diagnosing agenesis of the corpus callosum, and in viewing cortical malformations.[15,16] Areas that are not easily accessed by ultrasound, such as the posterior fossa, due to overlying bone, are better visualized on fetal MR imaging. MR imaging is very helpful in cystic malformations of the posterior fossa, in which it is better able than ultrasonography to detect whether dural structures, mostly tentorium, are normally positioned or not.[17] False-positive diagnosis of posterior fossa abnormalities have been reported by Poutamo and colleagues[18]; these are possibly caused by nonrecognition of the normal sequence of fetal brain development and normal variations in anatomy. Dandy-Walker malformation is characterized by an elevated tentorium, bulging of the parieto-occipital vault, and partial or total absence of vermis, whereas retrocerebellar pouch (Blake's pouch), which is part of the Dandy-Walker continuum, shows an elevated tentorium but a normal vermis (**Fig. 2**). By contrast, Chiari malformation has a small posterior fossa (**Fig. 3**). A normally positioned tentorium with a normal-sized posterior fossa is seen in other rare anomalies such as pontocerebellar hypoplasia, rhombencephalosynapsis, and rhombencephaloschizis.

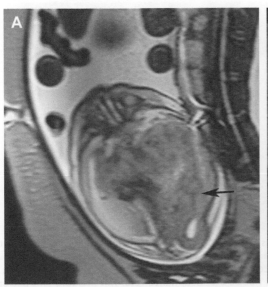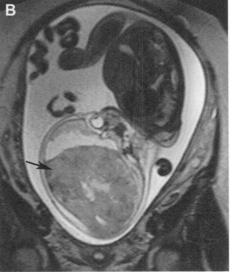

Fig. 7. Intracranial teratoma. Axial (A) and sagittal (B) T2-weighted images from a fetal MR image show a fetus with a large head due to a large intracranial mass (*arrow*). This involved bilateral cerebral hemispheres and led to bilateral ventriculomegaly. The mass was causing mass effect on the posterior cranial vault.

MR imaging is sensitive for intracranial hemorrhages (**Fig. 4**) and has been used in disorders such as alloimmune thrombocytopenia.[19] An early subacute bleed appears hyperintense on T1-weighted images and hypointense on T2-weighted images.[20] Hemoglobin can also be detected with gradient echo sequences that detect the signal loss caused by local magnetization of the iron in hemoglobin. Distinction between acute (1–3 days), early subacute (3–7 days), and late subacute (7–30 days) hemorrhages has not been reported in a fetus, and this is likely due to the difference between fetal and adult hemoglobin that would influence the appearance and accuracy of antenatal imaging of hemorrhage on MR imaging.[21]

MR imaging is very effective in assessing for additional findings in cases with absent cavum septum pellucidum (**Fig. 5**). Even though imaging

of the optic nerves is beyond the resolution of fetal MR imaging at present, MR imaging can help exclude other associated malformations such as schizencephaly (**Fig. 6**). Several conditions such as hypoxia, congenital infections, malformations, inherited inborn errors of metabolism, and tumors can lead to destruction of the fetal brain (**Fig. 7**). Diffusion and proton spectroscopy will help detect such cases.[22,23] Fetal intracranial neoplasms are rare and are often associated with polyhydramnios and hydrocephalus.[24]

MR imaging is not required for the diagnosis of neural tube defects because its incremental value is negligible in most cases. Ultrasonography is an effective method for identifying myelomeningocele and hindbrain malformations in most cases. There are conflicting reports of the advantages of MR imaging over ultrasonography,[25–27] but

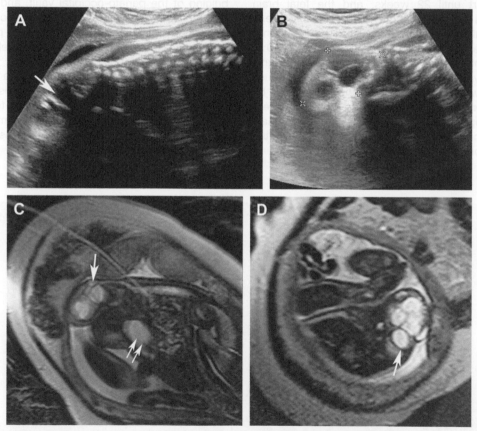

Fig. 8. Sacrococcygeal teratoma in a 32-week-old fetus. Ultrasound images in sagittal (*A*) and axial (*B*) orientation show a mixed solid cystic mass (*arrow* and *calipers*) arising from the sacrococcygeal region with internal vascularity consistent with a teratoma. Due to the advanced gestational age and ossification of the overlying bony structures, intra-abdominal extent of the mass could not be assessed; hence fetal MR imaging was performed. Sagittal oblique (*C*) and axial T2-weighted (*D*) images show a mixed solid cystic mass (*arrow*) in the sacrococcygeal region predominantly along the left gluteal region with no intra-abdominal extension. The mass is not seen to extend into or displace the bladder (*double arrows*).

MR imaging should certainly be performed if there is doubt regarding the diagnosis. In a study of 50 cases of suspected spinal cord abnormality, fetal MR findings differed from ultrasound findings in 10 cases, MR imaging correctly diagnosing normality or reclassifying the abnormality to one that was less severe, such as lipomyelomeningocele.[27] MR imaging is superior to ultrasonography in assessing sacrococcygeal teratomas, since these lesions can be incompletely assessed on ultrasonography because of shadowing from iliac and sacral bones.[28] Prognosis in sacrococcygeal teratoma depends on the degree of intra-abdominal extension, and this can be well evaluated by MR imaging, especially if fetal surgery is planned (**Fig. 8**).

MR imaging is evolving from providing an anatomic survey of anomalies to garnering functional information regarding fetal brain. Techniques such as diffusion-weighted imaging, proton spectroscopy, and functional imaging are being used for evaluation of fetal brain. Diffusion-weighted imaging is extensively used in the neonatal period to assess for hypoxic-induced damage, and it is hoped that these techniques can be used to diagnose impending ischemia before irreversible damage has occurred.

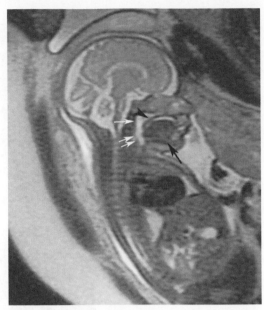

Fig. 9. Normal neck. Sagittal image through the fetus shows a normal appearance and location of the tongue (*black arrow*) and palate (*black arrowhead*). The nasopharynx (*white arrow*) and oropharynx (*double white arrow*) are also seen to be normal.

Head and Neck

Many congenital syndromes are associated with facial malformations. Because the fetus continuously swallows amniotic fluid, the naso- and oropharynx are usually fluid-filled and thus hyperintense on T2-weighted images (**Fig. 9**). MR imaging has proven to be particularly helpful in the assessment of patency of the fetal respiratory tract in fetuses with large neck masses such as lymphatic malformations (**Fig. 10**) and teratomas (**Fig. 11**).[29] Large neck masses can cause airway obstruction, leading to asphyxia and secondary brain damage if there is a long delay in securing an airway.[30] A planned delivery may also be necessary to optimize fetal outcome by using the EXIT procedure. However, because the EXIT procedure itself is associated with significant morbidity to the fetus and mother and potential mortality to the mother, careful prenatal assessment is essential. This workup can be achieved by using fetal MR imaging to assess the size and location of the mass and also evaluate the patency of the fetal respiratory tract.[31] Kuwashima and colleagues[32] have described a case of laryngeal atresia diagnosed at 24 weeks by MR imaging. Bilaterally enlarged high-signal lungs, dilated bronchi, massive ascites, subcutaneous edema, and polyhydramnios were seen on MR imaging, which helped them confirm the diagnosis.

Thyroid gland is usually indistinct on T2-weighted images, but appears hyperintense on T1-weighted images. A fetal goiter can hence be easily delineated.[33]

Chest

Normal fetal lung on T2-weighted images is homogeneous and has moderate signal intensity between that of the bright amniotic fluid and skeletal muscle. The thymus usually displays intermediate signal intensity, and the large vessels appear hypointense due to flow voids. Fetal MR imaging is very useful in the diagnosis of a diaphragmatic hernia, especially right-sided diaphragmatic hernias. Coronal and sagittal T2-weighted images are most useful for diagnosis of diaphragmatic hernia (**Fig. 12**). If a left-sided hernia is present, there is displacement of the stomach, the small bowel, and the colon into the chest, seen as T2 bright structures. Right-sided hernias, however, can be associated with a normal position of the stomach and are difficult to diagnose on ultrasonography. MR imaging is particularly helpful in these cases (**Fig. 13**). Because CDHs are associated with pulmonary hypoplasia, the degree of lung hypoplasia can be assessed by fetal MR imaging.[34] The lung volume can usually be easily estimated when imaging in

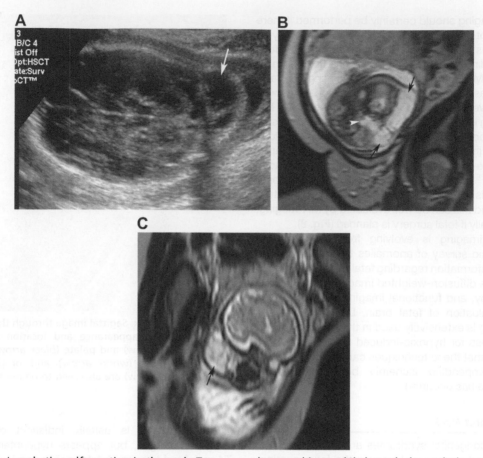

Fig. 10. Lymphatic malformation in the neck. Transverse ultrasound image (*A*) through the neck shows a cystic mass (*arrow*) predominantly in the posterolateral aspect of the neck. Axial (*B*) and sagittal (*C*) T2-weighted images show a predominantly cystic mass (*black arrow*) in the posterolateral neck with septations in it. This was a cystic lymphatic malformation with no extension into the chest or compression of the trachea; however, there was extension seen into the oral cavity along the lateral aspect (*arrowhead*).

3 planes has been performed and normal fetal lung volume is strongly correlated with biometric measurements.[35] Lung volumes were measured and expressed as a percentage of the predicted lung volume (PPLV) in a study by Barnewolt and colleagues.[36] Predicted lung volume was determined by subtracting measured mediastinal volume from total measured thoracic volume. The PPLV was correlated with postnatal outcomes. Of the 14 live-born patients, the PPLV was 20.3 ± 10.4. The PPLV was significantly associated with extracorporeal membrane oxygenation (ECMO) use, length of stay in hospital, and survival. All patients with a PPLV of less than 15 required prolonged ECMO support and had a 40% survival rate. By contrast, only 11% of patients with a PPLV of greater than 15 required ECMO, and survival was 100% in these cases. The investigators concluded that a PPLV value of

less than 15 is associated with a significantly higher risk for prolonged support and/or death, despite aggressive postnatal management. A study by Busing and colleagues[37,38] found similar results, suggesting that higher fetal lung volume was associated with improved survival (P<.001) and decreasing probability of need for ECMO therapy (P<.008). Axial T2-weighted MR images were used by Cannie and colleagues[39] to assess the degree of intrathoracic liver herniation by volumetry, using the xyphoid process and thoracic apex as landmarks. The ratio of the volume of the liver that was herniated into the thoracic cavity to the volume of the thoracic cavity was calculated. Assessment of ratio of the volume of the liver that was herniated into the thoracic cavity to the volume of the thoracic cavity using MR imaging provided prediction of postnatal survival independently of the total fetal lung volume. Studies

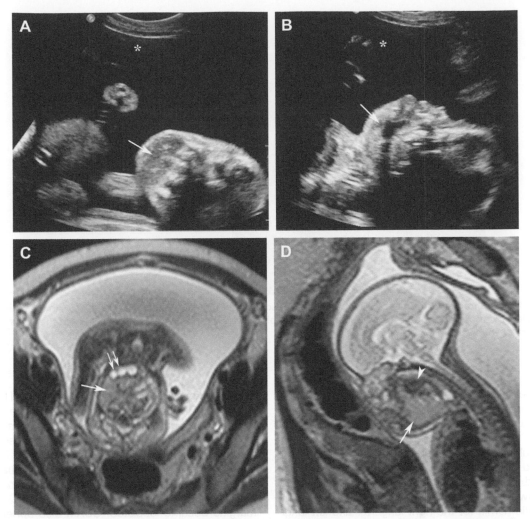

Fig. 11. Neck teratoma. Coronal (*A*) and sagittal (*B*) ultrasound images demonstrate a soft tissue mass in the floor of the mouth (*arrow*), which was difficult to easily discern. Note the associated severe polyhydramnios (*asterisk*). Fetal MR imaging (*C*, axial and *D*, sagittal images) reveals a large mass (*arrow*) in the floor of the mouth, displacing and invading the tongue (*arrowhead*) and causing obstruction of the oropharynx. Cystic areas were seen in the posterior aspect of this mass (*double arrow*). This was suggested to be a teratoma and was proven so on autopsy.

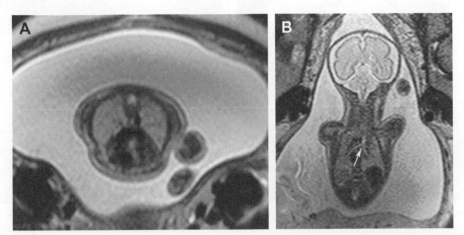

Fig. 12. Normal lungs. Normal appearance of the lungs on fetal MR imaging (*A*, axial and *B*, coronal). The high signal intensity is caused by fluid in the lungs. Note the tracheal bifurcation seen on the coronal image (*arrow*).

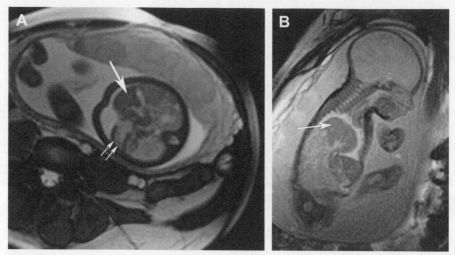

Fig. 13. Diaphragmatic hernia. T2-weighted axial (*A*) and sagittal (*B*) images show the liver (*arrow*) in the chest at the level of the heart (*double arrows*), suggesting a diaphragmatic hernia. Note the compression of the lungs and heart by the liver.

have been performed to evaluate the lungs by comparing the signal intensity of the lung to other organs. The hypothesis is that normal lungs are fluid filled; however, pulmonary hypoplasia would lead to a decrease in the amount of fluid in the lungs (**Fig. 14**). A study by Gorincour and colleagues[40] found significant differences between normal fetuses and fetuses with diaphragmatic hernia for the right lung/liver and left lung/psoas ratios.

In addition to CDHs, congenital cystic adenomatoid malformations (CCAM) and bronchopulmonary

sequestrations (BPS) can also be seen on fetal MR imaging.[33] BPS in the second trimester appear as well-defined, homogeneous, hyperintense masses (pure BPS) or as a lobulated, inhomogeneous hyperintense mass (BPS mixed with CCAM). The feeding artery can be seen. As the BPS mass regresses in the third trimester, the signal intensity decreases, becoming inhomogeneous, and the margins became lobulated. CCAM also appears as a hyperintense lobulated mass, and as the lesions regress they decrease in size and signal intensity. As with BPS, the larger the lesion on

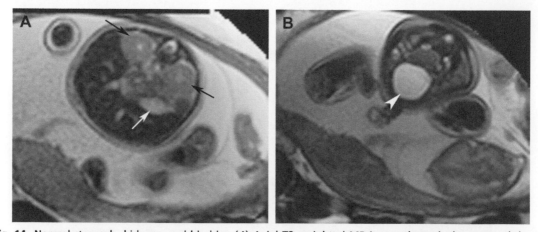

Fig. 14. Normal stomach, kidneys, and bladder. (*A*) Axial T2-weighted MR image through the upper abdomen shows normal appearance of the stomach seen as a fluid-filled structure in the left abdomen (*arrow*). Normal kidneys (*black arrows*) are seen posterior to the stomach. (*B*) Axial T2-weighted MR image through the pelvis shows the bladder (*arrowhead*) seen as a cystic structure.

initial MR imaging, the less likely it is to regress completely. Congenital lobar fluid overload appears as a hyperintense, homogeneous lobe with stretched hilar vessels.[41] Fetal cardiac imaging cannot be performed at the current state of technology. Fetal cardiac triggering is not feasible in most instances, and the resolution of the cardiac chambers remains suboptimal.

Gastrointestinal Tract

Gastrointestinal anomalies account for a small proportion of cases imaged by fetal MR imaging. As the fetus swallows the amniotic fluid, it serves as a natural "contrast agent" on T2-weighted sequences. The fluid-filled stomach and proximal small bowel loops appear hyperintense (see **Fig. 14**) on T2-weighted images; however, the distal small bowel loops and the colon are generally hypointense on T2-weighted and hyperintense on T1-weighted images, because they contain the more viscous meconium.[42] Duodenal atresia, small bowel atresia, and malrotation can be recognized on fetal MR imaging.[43] The liver is seen in the normal right subdiaphragmatic location, and the adjacent gallbladder should be fluid-filled and thus hyperintense on T2-weighted images. Congenital liver masses include infantile hemangioblastomas (**Fig. 15**), hepatoblastomas, cysts, hemangiomas, and mesenchymal hamartomas.[44] Spleen appears isointense to the liver, and absence of the spleen can help diagnose

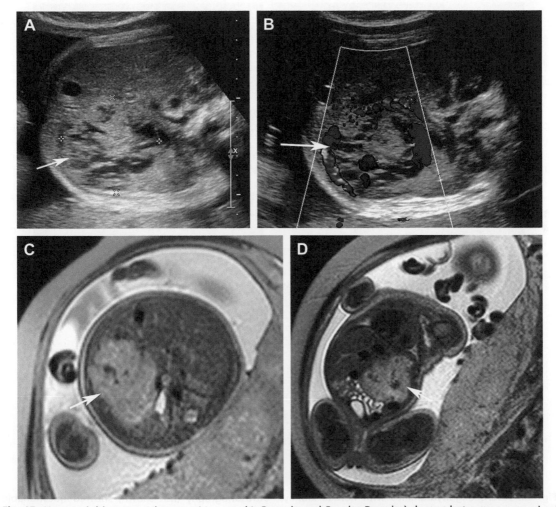

Fig. 15. Hemangioblastoma. Ultrasound images (*A*, B-mode and *B*, color Doppler) show a heterogeneous mixed solid and cystic mass (*arrow*) in the left lobe of the liver in a 32-week-old fetus. This was suspected to be a hemangioblastoma. Fetal MR imaging (*C, D*) confirmed the findings with large high signal intensity mass (*arrow*) in the left lobe with prominent flow voids caused by high flow.

heterotaxy syndromes. Abdominal wall defects are usually well seen on ultrasonography; however, MR imaging can help in the diagnosis of complex lesions and in identifying associated anomalies and contents of the hernia. MR imaging can be more accurate in diagnosing bowel lesions such as small bowel atresia, which is seen as dilated bowel loops proximal to the obstruction.[45] MR imaging has been used in patients with suspected meconium peritonitis as well, and the presence of normal bowel or the location of atretic bowel can be assessed. Pseudocysts seen in meconium peritonitis have a fluid-like signal on T2-weighted images; however, the signal intensity on T1-weighted images is intermediate, which is different from that seen in intestinal duplication, which has low signal intensity on T1-weighted images.[45]

Urogenital System

The urogenital system is involved in 0.1% of congenital disorders. As the fetus swallows amniotic fluid, urine is continuously being produced. A fluid-filled bladder is an indirect sign of a functioning renal excretory system. The kidneys themselves should also be scrutinized for malformations (**Fig. 16**). Various causes of hydronephrosis such as ureteropelvic junction obstruction, ureterovesicular junction obstruction,

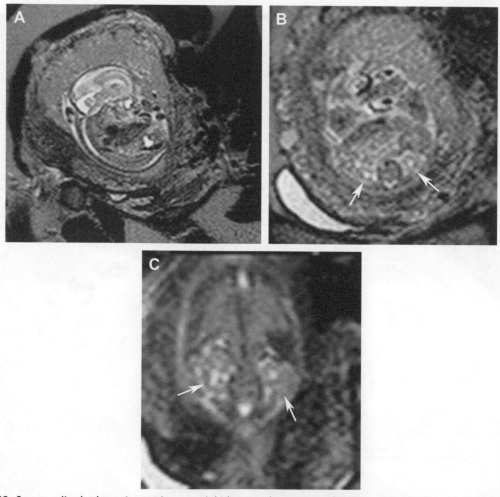

Fig. 16. Severe oligohydramnios with normal kidneys. Ultrasonography (not shown) showed questionable presence of bilateral kidneys along with severe oligohydramnios. Fetal MR imaging was performed, which again showed the severe oligohydramnios (note lack of fluid around the fetus on sagittal image [*A*]). Axial (*B*) and coronal (*C*) images through the abdomen show presence and normal appearance of bilateral kidneys (*arrows*).

and posterior urethral valves can be diagnosed.[46] The spectrum of malformations is wide, and prognosis depends on the presence or absence of bilateral lesions and oligohydramnios (see **Fig. 16**). MR imaging evaluates well the various forms of cystic kidneys such as multicystic dysplastic kidneys and autosomal recessive polycystic kidneys, especially when the diagnosis is not confirmed on ultrasonography.[47] Bilateral agenesis or hypogenesis can be differentiated with certainty from an ectopic location of the kidneys. The gender of a male fetus can be easily

noted on sagittal MR images; however, female external genitalia are difficult to discern (**Fig. 17**).

Musculoskeletal System

The most commonly encountered pathologic entity of the limbs is arthrogryposis multiplex (**Fig. 18**). The lack of fluid, CNS abnormality and syndromes such as Pena-Shokeir result in arthrogryposis. Malpositioning of the extremities leads to eventual shortening of the tendons and deformation of the distal extremities. Ultrasonography is essential in

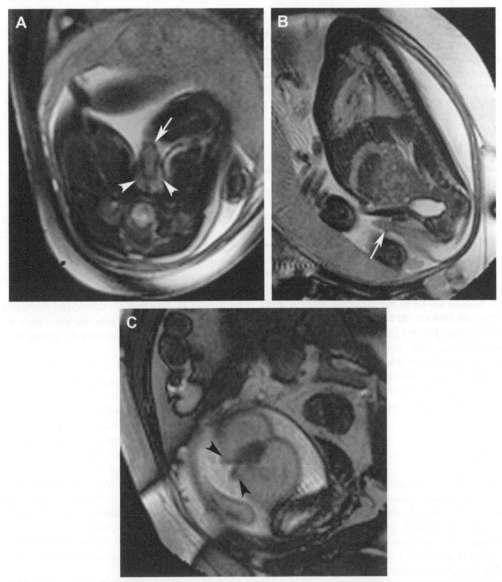

Fig. 17. Normal genitalia. Axial T2-weighted (*A*) and sagittal T2-weighted (*B*) MR images show normal male genitalia with penile shaft (*arrow*) and scrotal sacs (*arrowheads*). Axial T2-weighted image (*C*) in a female fetus shows normal female genitalia with labial folds seen bilaterally (*black arrowheads*).

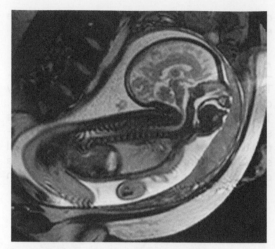

Fig. 18. Arthrogryposis. Abnormal positioning of the fetus is seen on T2-weighted sagittal MR image as a persistent hyperextension of the neck with crossing of the arms and fingers in a fetus with arthrogryposis. There was relative paucity of musculature in the fetal arms and legs as well (not shown).

assessing the fetal movement in these cases; however, fetal MR imaging can be used to evaluate the fetal CNS in these cases.[48]

SUMMARY

Fetal MR imaging has become instrumental in the management of complicated fetal anomalies. Although ultrasonography will and should remain the method of choice for prenatal screening, MR imaging should be used for complex lesions and indeterminate lesions discerned on an ultrasonogram. MR imaging is now being used more regularly for prenatal diagnosis, counseling, and management planning of fetal anomalies. Knowledge of the techniques available for MR imaging of fetuses with normal anatomy and the limitations of fetal MR imaging are essential for radiologists and obstetricians alike.

REFERENCES

1. Smith F, Adam A, Phillips W. NMR imaging in pregnancy. Lancet 1983;1(8314-5):61-2.
2. Santos X, Papanna R, Johnson A, et al. The use of combined ultrasound and magnetic resonance imaging in the detection of fetal anomalies. Prenat Diagn 2010;30(5):402-7.
3. Baker P, Johnson I, Harvey P, et al. A three-year follow-up of children imaged in utero with echo-planar magnetic resonance. Am J Obstet Gynecol 1994;170(1 Pt 1):32-3.
4. Kanal E, Gillen J, Evans J, et al. Survey of reproductive health among female MR workers. Radiology 1993;187(2):395-9.
5. National Radiological Protection Board. Principles for the protection of patients and volunteers during clinical magnetic resonance diagnostic procedures: documents of the NRPB. London: HM Stationery Office; 1991.
6. Shellock F, Kanal E. Policies, guidelines, and recommendations for MR imaging safety and patient management. SMRI Safety Committee. J Magn Reson Imaging 1991;1(1):97-101.
7. Glover P, Hykin J, Gowland P, et al. An assessment of the intrauterine sound intensity level during obstetric echo-planar magnetic resonance imaging. Br J Radiol 1995;68(814):1090-4.
8. Chung H, Chen C, Zimmerman R, et al. T2-Weighted fast MR imaging with true FISP versus HASTE: comparative efficacy in the evaluation of normal fetal brain maturation. AJR Am J Roentgenol 2000; 175(5):1375-80.
9. Ertl-Wagner B, Lienemann A, Strauss A, et al. Fetal magnetic resonance imaging: indications, technique, anatomical considerations and a review of fetal abnormalities. Eur Radiol 2002;12(8):1931-40.
10. Levine D, Barnes P, Robertson R, et al. Fast MR imaging of fetal central nervous system abnormalities. Radiology 2003;229(1):51-61.
11. Twickler D, Magee K, Caire J, et al. Second-opinion magnetic resonance imaging for suspected fetal central nervous system abnormalities. Am J Obstet Gynecol 2003;188(2):492-6.
12. Levine D, Barnes P. Cortical maturation in normal and abnormal fetuses as assessed with prenatal MR imaging. Radiology 1999;210(3):751-8.
13. Girard N, Raybaud C. Ventriculomegaly and pericerebral CSF collection in the fetus: early stage of benign external hydrocephalus? Childs Nerv Syst 2001;17(4/5):239-45.
14. Benacerraf B, Shipp T, Bromley B, et al. What does magnetic resonance imaging add to the prenatal sonographic diagnosis of ventriculomegaly? J Ultrasound Med 2007;26(11):1513-22.
15. d'Ercole C, Girard N, Cravello L, et al. Prenatal diagnosis of fetal corpus callosum agenesis by ultrasonography and magnetic resonance imaging. Prenat Diagn 1998;18(3):247-53.
16. Glenn O, Barkovich A. Magnetic resonance imaging of the fetal brain and spine: an increasingly important tool in prenatal diagnosis, part 1. AJNR Am J Neuroradiol 2006;27(8):1604-11.
17. Raybaud C, Levrier O, Brunel H, et al. MR imaging of fetal brain malformations. Childs Nerv Syst 2003; 19(7/8):455-70.
18. Poutamo J, Vanninen R, Partanen K, et al. Magnetic resonance imaging supplements ultrasonographic imaging of the posterior fossa, pharynx and neck

in malformed fetuses. Ultrasound Obstet Gynecol 1999;13(5):327–34.

19. Dale S, Coleman L. Neonatal alloimmune thrombocytopenia: antenatal and postnatal imaging findings in the pediatric brain. AJNR Am J Neuroradiol 2002; 23(9):1457–65.

20. Canapicchi R, Cioni G, Strigini F, et al. Prenatal diagnosis of periventricular hemorrhage by fetal brain magnetic resonance imaging. Childs Nerv Syst 1998; 14(12):689–92.

21. Brugger P, Stuhr F, Lindner C, et al. Methods of fetal MR: beyond T2-weighted imaging. Eur J Radiol 2006; 57(2):172–81.

22. Brunel H, Girard N, Confort-Gouny S, et al. Fetal brain injury. J Neuroradiol 2004;31(2):123–37.

23. Girard N, Fogliarini C, Viola A, et al. MRS of normal and impaired fetal brain development. Eur J Radiol 2006;57(2):217–25.

24. Cavalheiro S, Moron A, Zymberg S, et al. Fetal hydrocephalus—prenatal treatment. Childs Nerv Syst 2003; 19(7/8):561–73.

25. Aaronson O, Hernanz-Schulman M, Bruner J, et al. Myelomeningocele: prenatal evaluation—comparison between transabdominal US and MR imaging. Radiology 2003;227(3):839–43.

26. Mangels K, Tulipan N, Tsao L, et al. Fetal MRI in the evaluation of intrauterine myelomeningocele. Pediatr Neurosurg 2000;32(3):124–31.

27. Griffiths P, Widjaja E, Paley M, et al. Imaging the fetal spine using in utero MR: diagnostic accuracy and impact on management. Pediatr Radiol 2006;36(9): 927–33.

28. Avni F, Guibaud L, Robert Y, et al. MR imaging of fetal sacrococcygeal teratoma: diagnosis and assessment. AJR Am J Roentgenol 2002;178(1):179–83.

29. Kathary N, Bulas D, Newman K, et al. MRI imaging of fetal neck masses with airway compromise: utility in delivery planning. Pediatr Radiol 2001;31(10):727–31.

30. Mychaliska G, Bealer J, Graf J, et al. Operating on placental support: the ex utero intrapartum treatment procedure. J Pediatr Surg 1997;32(2):227–30 [discussion: 230–1].

31. Hubbard A, Crombleholme T, Adzick N. Prenatal MRI evaluation of giant neck masses in preparation for the fetal exit procedure. Am J Perinatol 1998;15(4):253–7.

32. Kuwashima S, Kitajima K, Kaji Y, et al. MR imaging appearance of laryngeal atresia (congenital high airway obstruction syndrome): unique course in a fetus. Pediatr Radiol 2008;38(3):344–7.

33. Shinmoto H, Kashima K, Yuasa Y, et al. MR imaging of non-CNS fetal abnormalities: a pictorial essay. Radiographics 2000;20(5):1227–43.

34. Paek B, Coakley F, Lu Y, et al. Congenital diaphragmatic hernia: prenatal evaluation with MR lung volumetry—preliminary experience. Radiology 2001;220(1):63–7.

35. Coakley F, Lopoo J, Lu Y, et al. Normal and hypoplastic fetal lungs: volumetric assessment with prenatal single-shot rapid acquisition with relaxation enhancement MR imaging. Radiology 2000;216(1): 107–11.

36. Barnewolt C, Kunisaki S, Fauza D, et al. Percent predicted lung volumes as measured on fetal magnetic resonance imaging: a useful biometric parameter for risk stratification in congenital diaphragmatic hernia. J Pediatr Surg 2007;42(1):193–7.

37. Büsing K, Kilian A, Schaible T, et al. MR lung volume in fetal congenital diaphragmatic hernia: logistic regression analysis—mortality and extracorporeal membrane oxygenation. Radiology 2008;248(1): 233–9.

38. Büsing K, Kilian A, Schaible T, et al. MR relative fetal lung volume in congenital diaphragmatic hernia: survival and need for extracorporeal membrane oxygenation. Radiology 2008;248(1):240–6.

39. Cannie M, Jani J, Meersschaert J, et al. Prenatal prediction of survival in isolated diaphragmatic hernia using observed to expected total fetal lung volume determined by magnetic resonance imaging based on either gestational age or fetal body volume. Ultrasound Obstet Gynecol 2008;32(5):633–9.

40. Gorincour G, Bach-Segura P, Ferry-Juquin M, et al. Lung signal on fetal MRI: normal values and usefulness for congenital diaphragmatic hernia. J Radiol 2009;90(1 Pt 1):53–8 [in French].

41. Liu Y, Chen C, Shih S, et al. Fetal cystic lung lesions: evaluation with magnetic resonance imaging. Pediatr Pulmonol 2010;45(6):592–600.

42. Hubbard A, Harty P. Prenatal magnetic resonance imaging of fetal anomalies. Semin Roentgenol 1999; 34(1):41–7.

43. Biyyam D, Dighe M, Siebert J. Antenatal diagnosis of intestinal malrotation on fetal MRI. Pediatr Radiol 2009;39(8):847–9.

44. Brunelle F, Chaumont P. Hepatic tumors in children: ultrasonic differentiation of malignant from benign lesions. Radiology 1984;150(3):695–9.

45. Veyrac C, Couture A, Saguintaah M, et al. MRI of fetal GI tract abnormalities. Abdom Imaging 2004; 29(4):411–20.

46. Guys J, Borella F, Monfort G. Ureteropelvic junction obstructions: prenatal diagnosis and neonatal surgery in 47 cases. J Pediatr Surg 1988;23(2):156–8.

47. Cassart M, Massez A, Metens T, et al. Complementary role of MRI after sonography in assessing bilateral urinary tract anomalies in the fetus. AJR Am J Roentgenol 2004;182(3):689–95.

48. Senocak E, Oguz K, Haliloglu G, et al. Prenatal diagnosis of Pena-Shokeir syndrome phenotype by ultrasonography and MR imaging. Pediatr Radiol 2009; 39(4):377–80.

Imaging of the Pregnant Patient for Nonobstetric Conditions

Puneet Bhargava, MBBS, DNB[a,b,*]

KEYWORDS

• Imaging appropriateness • Pregnancy • Radiation risks

Radiologists should be well aware of the published evidence of risks of radiation to the fetus because imaging of pregnant women is often required in the clinical workup. It has been demonstrated that the awareness of radiation risks associated with pregnant women is lower than expected.[1,2] The practice patterns at various institutions vary slightly because of the availability of various resources, and radiologists are best suited to optimize the imaging protocol. The protocol is planned in consensus with the clinical team and targeted at the clinical scenario. Risk versus benefit should be carefully considered, and an informed consent from the patient should be obtained. When radiation cannot be avoided, the conventional imaging protocols should be altered to achieve the lowest exposure. However, there is a lack of sufficient evidence in the literature that a single imaging study is certainly harmful to the fetus. Radiation dose to the fetus can be estimated using fetal dosimetry, and a medical physicist should be consulted when available. No imaging study, including an interventional procedure, should be avoided or deferred when a delay in the diagnosis could potentially harm the pregnant woman or the fetus.[3]

It is considered good practice to obtain informed consent from the patient regarding the use of imaging modality and contrast agents. It is important to document that risk versus benefit of performing the studies was considered, risk of radiation exposure to the fetus was explained,

and alternatives were discussed, including the use of alternate modalities and risks associated with not performing any imaging study.

This article reviews the common imaging scenarios in pregnancy that may warrant imaging, with the exception of trauma by Claudia Sadro, which is considered as a separate topic in this issue.

RADIATION EFFECTS

Risks of radiation can be characterized as stochastic and nonstochastic effects. Stochastic effects are independent of the radiation dose, have no threshold value, and can occur with any amount of ionizing radiation. These effects are the result of cellular damage at the DNA level, causing cancer or other germ cell mutations. Radiation dose estimated for stochastic effects has been established at 50 mGy (ie, 5 rad).[4] In 2008, the American College of Radiology (ACR) published practice guidelines for imaging the pregnant woman and provided the estimated fetal risk at various gestational ages with differing radiation exposure. Theoretical risks were shown to be present only at doses higher than 100 mGy (10 rad).[5]

Nonstochastic or deterministic effects are predictable and caused at higher doses, and they involve chromosomal aberrations. A threshold dose of 150 mGy (15 rad) is reported.[6] Risks at this dose, again theoretical estimates, include a less than 3% chance of cancer development,

The author has nothing to disclose.
[a] Department of Radiology, University of Washington, 1959 NE Pacific Street, BB 308, Seattle, WA 98195, USA
[b] Diagnostic Imaging Services, Veterans Affairs Puget Sound Health Care System, 1660 South Columbian Way, S-114/Radiology, Seattle, WA 98108, USA
* Diagnostic Imaging Services, Veterans Affairs Puget Sound Health Care System, 1660 South Columbian Way, S-114/Radiology, Seattle, WA 98108.
E-mail address: bhargp@u.washington.edu

Ultrasound Clin 6 (2011) 87–95
doi:10.1016/j.cult.2010.11.001
1556-858X/11/$ – see front matter. Published by Elsevier Inc.

a 6% chance of mental retardation, loss of IQ points by 30 points per 100 mGy, and a 15% chance of microcephaly.[3,7–9]

An average single imaging study exposes the fetus to much less than 50 mGy (5 rad). Thus the concern for fetal radiation should not delay imaging studies.[3]

CHOICE OF MODALITY AND USE OF CONTRAST

Planning of an imaging study revolves around the choice of modality to be used. In general, ultrasonography (US) should always be the initial modality for evaluation, and the other modalities are used only if the results of US are inconclusive, especially in the first trimester.[3,5] Magnetic resonance (MR) imaging has the advantages of lack of ionizing radiation, multiplanar capability, and excellent soft tissue contrast.[3,10] Although there is a lack of controlled studies, the risk to the fetus at 1.5-T magnetic field strength is considered negligible, and safety at higher field strengths has not been assessed.[3,11] Often MR imaging is unavailable or inaccessible at short notice, and radiation exposure cannot be avoided. In 1991, the Safety Committee of the Society of Magnetic Resonance Imaging stated that "MR imaging may be used in pregnant women if other non-ionizing forms of diagnostic imaging are inadequate or if diagnosis would otherwise require exposure to ionizing radiation. Pregnant patients should be informed that, to date, there has been no indication that the use of clinical MR imaging during pregnancy has produced deleterious effects."[3,12]

Use of computed tomography (CT), plain radiography, and fluoroscopy is associated with radiation exposure, and these modalities should be used with caution. CT should be performed using low-dose protocols. The estimated radiation exposure is low for CT when the fetus is outside the field of view. Radiation dose is of most concern after multiple consecutive studies have been performed and accumulated radiation dose reaches the threshold dose.[3] ACR guidelines emphasize on using the ALARA (as low as reasonably achievable) principle and performing studies after careful consideration of risk versus benefit.

Oral contrast is not considered as a threat to pregnant patients, and intraluminal barium may, in fact, act as internal shielding.[11] Intravenous iodinated contrast crosses the placenta and enters the fetus in clinical doses.[3,11] No mutagenic or teratogenic effects with low-osmolality contrast media have been seen in animal studies.[3,10,11] However, given the concern for damage to fetal thyroid gland from iodine uptake, thyroid function should be checked in the first few weeks of life if the mother had received iodinated contrast during pregnancy.[3,11] Gadolinium-based contrast agents also cross the placenta in clinical doses, but no direct toxic effects have been shown in humans. The Committee on Drugs and Contrast Media recommends that radiologists confer with the referring physician and discuss the potential clinical benefit of MR imaging compared with that of other modalities and the necessity of gadolinium for diagnosis.[13] However, gadolinium is a class C drug, and its safety in humans is not established.[3]

CLINICAL SCENARIOS
Pulmonary Embolism

Pregnant women are at an increased risk for deep vein thrombosis by a factor of 5, and venous thromboembolism is a leading cause of maternal mortality.[3,14] Venous thromboembolism is attributed to an increased severity of venous stasis as well as the hypercoagulable state associated with pregnancy. A pregnant woman with a diagnosis of pulmonary embolism may need to consider prophylactic anticoagulation in future pregnancies and avoid the use of oral contraceptives. It is thus imperative to diagnose or exclude pulmonary embolism in pregnant patients if there is a clinical suspicion.[11] In a pregnant woman, D-dimer assay is mainly performed to obtain its negative predictive value because the D-dimer levels are usually elevated during pregnancy.[3,11,14,15] The threshold levels of normal D-dimer in different trimesters are yet to be established, thus imaging has to be relied on to diagnose or exclude pulmonary embolism.[11,16]

A chest radiograph with lead shielding of the abdomen along with vascular US of the lower extremity veins should be performed as an initial study, and if a positive result is obtained, it can obviate further workup. Because the treatment of deep vein thrombosis and pulmonary embolism is the same, a positive US result avoids additional imaging.[11] The limitations of compression US include lack of studies validating the above-mentioned recommendation and its low sensitivity for iliac vein thrombosis, which is more common in pregnant patients than in nonpregnant patients.[11,17] If US results are negative or inconclusive and the clinical suspicion remains high, CT pulmonary angiography should be performed (**Fig. 1**).[3,10,18–20]

The choice of imaging studies includes a CT pulmonary angiography and a ventilation/perfusion (V/Q) scan. CT pulmonary angiography is the study of choice because although it has radiation exposure similar to that of a V/Q scan, it is more likely

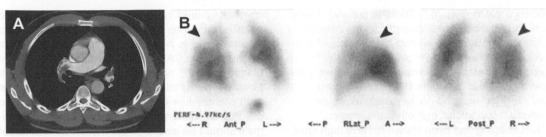

Fig. 1. Pulmonary embolism in 2 pregnant patients. (A) Bilateral pulmonary emboli in a 36-year-old woman in the first trimester with a history of worsening shortness of breath. Axial contrast-enhanced CT image shows bilateral pulmonary emboli. (B) Segmental pulmonary embolus in a 34-year-old woman in the first trimester with a history of worsening shortness of breath, normal chest radiographic findings, and a severe allergy to iodinated contrast material. Images from a ventilation-perfusion scintigraphic study show a mismatch in the right upper lobe (arrowhead) due to a segmental pulmonary embolus. (Reproduced from Wieseler KM, Bhargava P, Kanal KM, et al. Imaging in pregnant patients: examination appropriateness. Radiographics 2010;30:1215–9; with permission.)

to identify the cause of chest pain when the underlying diagnosis is not pulmonary embolism.[3,14,19] It also has a higher sensitivity (81%–91%) and specificity (93%–97%) than V/Q scanning for the detection of main, lobar, and segmental pulmonary arteries. The sensitivity of a high-probability V/Q scan is only 41%.[11,15] Radiation exposure to the fetus is limited and scatter radiation to the uterus is small when CT is performed in the first and early second trimesters. There is a potential increased risk of maternal radiation-induced breast cancer with CT angiography.[11,16,21] V/Q scan is the study of choice if there is allergy to iodinated contrast material. The classic finding in a study that is positive for pulmonary embolism is mismatched perfusion defects. A negative V/Q scan result can exclude the diagnosis of pulmonary embolism with a negative predictive value of close to 100% but is unlikely to define the cause of chest pain.[3,22] The algorithm used at the author's institution for imaging a pregnant patient suspected of having a pulmonary embolism is shown in **Fig. 2**.

Appendicitis

The appendix is the most common cause of surgical abdomen in pregnancy.[3] Appendicitis in a pregnant patient is associated with premature labor, fetal morbidity and mortality, and a higher rate of perforation (43% vs 4%–19% in the general population).[11,23,24] Clinical signs of appendicitis, such as right lower quadrant pain, nausea, vomiting, and leukocytosis, are not reliable in pregnancy, and the delay in diagnosis contributes to a higher risk of perforation.[11,24] The appendix is also displaced by the gravid uterus.[25,26] US with graded compression technique is the first-line imaging because of the lack of ionizing radiation and its ability to survey the pelvis for alternate diagnoses, but the appendix is not visualized in up to 88% to 92% of examinations.[11,25,27–29] The

appendix may be difficult to localize in patients more than 15 weeks pregnant and in those with body mass index (BMI, calculated as the weight in kilograms divided by height in meters squared) of more than 30.[3] In the third trimester, visualization is improved when the patient is imaged in the left lateral decubitus position.[11,27] US findings in acute appendicitis include a blind-ending tubular structure larger than 6 mm with thick hyperemic walls, inflammatory fat stranding, and

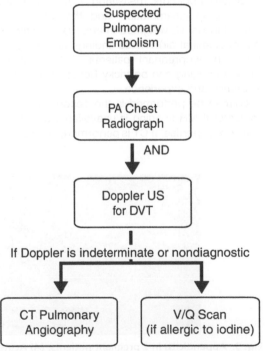

Fig. 2. Algorithm for workup of suspected pulmonary embolism in a pregnant patient. DVT, deep venous thrombosis; PA, posteroanterior. (Reproduced from Wieseler KM, Bhargava P, Kanal KM, et al. Imaging in pregnant patients: examination appropriateness. Radiographics 2010;30:1215–9; with permission.)

appendicoliths (**Fig. 3**).[30] There is superior migration and rotation of the appendix as the pregnancy advances. US is also limited by operator dependence, presence of bowel gas, and obesity. Therefore, if US results are negative or indeterminate and a definitive alternate diagnosis is not identified, further imaging is required to confirm or exclude appendicitis and other diagnoses.[11,31]

MR imaging has been shown to have high specificity and sensitivity for the detection of appendicitis and other abdominal and pelvic pathologic conditions in pregnant patients with acute right lower quadrant abdominal pain.[11] It should be performed when US is unable to show the appendix, the fetus is beyond 15 weeks' gestation, and the patient's BMI is more than 30.[3] Recent review of the literature suggests that MR imaging can visualize the appendix in 87% to 100% of cases.[29,32,33] The negative predictive value of MR imaging for the diagnosis of appendicitis has been reported at 100%.[25,28] Negative contrast oral agents, such as a mixture of ferumoxsil and barium sulfate, may be used to decrease susceptibility artifacts and improve the identification of a fluid-filled appendix.[26] Single-shot fast spin-echo images are obtained to decrease artifacts from peristalsis, and findings typically include a dilated appendix measuring 7 mm or more, surrounding inflammation, and the absence of blooming on T2-weighted images (suggestive of no intraluminal air). These findings are similar to those in nonpregnant patients.[3,26,34] Diagnosis on MR imaging can be tricky because of lack of expertise and experience.

CT can be performed in the second and third trimester if MR imaging is unavailable or there is a lack of expertise. If CT is performed, intravenous contrast should be used unless contraindicated because of iodine allergy.[3,11] Oral contrast should also be used to help improve the visualization of the appendix.[11] Although the risk of delaying the diagnosis of appendicitis with subsequent possible perforation outweighs the concern of the potential risk of developing radiation-induced childhood concern, both clinicians and radiologists should be aware of the theoretical risk associated with the study (ie, approximately 1 case with cancer per 500 fetuses exposed to 30 mGy).[11,35] This information should be used to encourage more avid efforts to keep the radiation dose as low as possible (eg, by decreasing the milliampere-seconds value, using z-axis modulation, and increasing the pitch).[11] Practice patterns can vary among various institutions, but CT should not be withheld or deferred if appendicitis remains the clinical concern because of high associated maternal mortality. The algorithm used at the author's institution for imaging pregnant patients suspected of having appendicitis is shown in **Fig. 4**.

Nonspecific Abdominal Pain

Localizing the source of abdominal pain in a pregnant woman is always a challenge because of the displacement of organs by the gravid uterus. Diseases of the liver, gall bladder, pancreas, bowel, including the appendix, pancreas, urinary tract, and ovary, can all present with nonspecific abdominal pain.[3] Abdominal US is the preferred initial examination and may identify the pathologic condition. Dilated bowel loops may suggest ileus, and focal abnormalities may direct focused

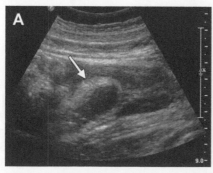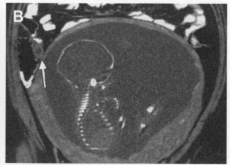

Fig. 3. Appendicitis in 2 pregnant patients. (*A*) Acute appendicitis in a 35-year-old patient in the third trimester with a history of nausea, vomiting, fever, and abdominal pain. US image shows an enlarged, dilated, tubular structure measuring 10 mm in diameter in the right lower quadrant (*arrow*), a finding suggestive of acute appendicitis. (*B*) Acute appendicitis in a 28-year-old woman in the third trimester with a history of acute pain in the right lower quadrant. Coronal contrast-enhanced reformatted CT image shows an enlarged appendix measuring 9 mm in diameter (*arrow*). (*Reproduced from* Wieseler KM, Bhargava P, Kanal KM, et al. Imaging in pregnant patients: examination appropriateness. Radiographics 2010;30:1215–9; with permission.)

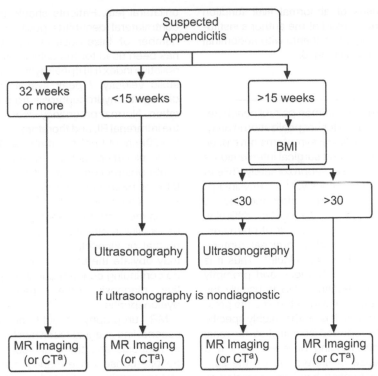

Fig. 4. Algorithm for workup of right lower quadrant abdominal pain in a pregnant patient when there is a strong suspicion of appendicitis. [a] Use CT if MR imaging is unavailable. (*Reproduced from* Wieseler KM, Bhargava P, Kanal KM, et al. Imaging in pregnant patients: examination appropriateness. Radiographics 2010;30:1215–9; with permission.)

evaluation of a quadrant in the abdomen. MR imaging may be performed as the second-line study.

CT scans using low-dose protocols can provide excellent information in a nonpregnant patient, with minimal radiation exposure.[3,25,33,36] Use of contrast may be required depending on the clinical scenario. CT enterography is especially useful in the diagnosis of Crohn disease in which the findings correlate with the stage of the disease. In the active inflammatory state, it can show wall thickening, hyperenhancement, mural stratification, reactive stranding in the mesenteric fat, and engorged vasa recta (comb sign). In the fibrostenotic variant, CT can show areas of strictures and fistula (Fig. 5).[3,37,38] Symptomatic biliary tract disease in pregnancy is uncommon. US is the initial study of choice. There is an increasing trend toward surgical management of biliary colic and acute cholecystitis in pregnancy, and complications, such as obstructive jaundice, gall stone pancreatitis, and peritonitis, are associated with high maternal and fetal mortality.[11,39,40] If US results are inconclusive, then MR cholangiopancreatography should be performed. It has a high sensitivity (98%) and specificity (84%) for diagnosis of biliary disease.[41] MR cholangiopancreatography is comparable to

endoscopic retrograde cholangiopancreatography (ERCP) for the diagnosis of choledocholithiasis, and ERCP should be reserved for those patients who need interventions.[11,42] MR imaging can also

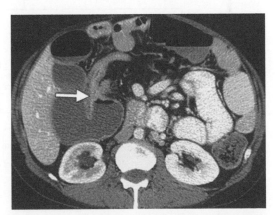

Fig. 5. Crohn disease in a 34-year-old patient in the second trimester with nausea, vomiting, and abdominal pain. Axial contrast-enhanced CT images show a stricture in the proximal small bowel (*arrow*) with proximal obstruction, mucosal enhancement, and fibrofatty proliferation in the surrounding mesentery. (*Reproduced from* Wieseler KM, Bhargava P, Kanal KM, et al. Imaging in pregnant patients: examination appropriateness. Radiographics 2010;30:1215–9; with permission.)

depict other causes of abnormal liver function tests.[11] The algorithm used at the author's institution for imaging pregnant patients with abdominal or pelvic pain is shown in **Fig. 6**.

Urolithiasis

Urolithiasis is the most common painful nonobstetric condition and reason for hospitalization in pregnant patients.[11,43,44] Clinical symptoms have been shown to be unreliable, and surgical intervention is not needed in most cases; approximately 75% of the calculi pass spontaneously.[3,11,45] Physiologic hydronephrosis of pregnancy after the second trimester also poses a diagnostic difficulty. However, there is an increased risk of premature labor induced by renal colic, forniceal rupture, and pyelonephritis with renal calculi.[11] Thus it is imperative to accurately diagnose and promptly treat urolithiasis in pregnancy. US is usually the first-line imaging and useful to determine the presence of hydronephrosis. It is neither highly specific nor sensitive, with reported sensitivities for renal and ureteric calculi ranging between 34% and 95%.[44,46,47] Absence of ureteral jet on the suspected side of obstruction has been reported to have a sensitivity of 100% and specificity of 91%.[48] Approximately 15% of asymptomatic pregnant women have been reported to have absent

unilateral jets. Patients should be imaged in the contralateral decubitus position to decrease the number of false-positive results.[49] Doppler US has been used for the calculation of the intrarenal resistive index (RI) ([peak systolic velocity - end diastolic velocity] / peak systolic velocity) to help distinguish hydronephrosis from physiologic dilatation. Normal pregnancy does not usually affect the intrarenal RI, and therefore, an elevated RI value (>0.70) should not be attributed to pregnancy. RI value elevation usually occurs within 6 hours of acute obstruction, and a difference in RI value of 0.04 or more between the normal and abnormal kidneys may be useful.[11,50,51] A transvaginal US is recommended to detect distal ureteral calculi, especially if results of transabdominal US are normal or inconclusive.[11,52] A normal sonogram may obviate the use of further imaging if there is no continuing concern about a significant alternative diagnosis other than renal colic or pyelonephritis.[11]

MR urography should be considered the second-line imaging test when US fails to establish a diagnosis and there are continued symptoms despite conservative management. Limitations of MR urography are limited visualization of smaller calculi and relatively high cost.[11] High sensitivity has been reported for the detection of urinary tract dilatation and identification of the site of

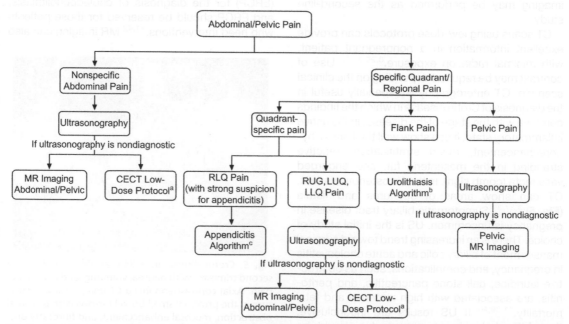

Fig. 6. Algorithm for workup of abdominal or pelvic pain in a pregnant patient. CECT, contrast-enhanced CT; LLQ, left lower quadrant; LUQ, left upper quadrant; RLQ, right lower quadrant; RUQ, right upper quadrant. [a] Use if MR imaging is unavailable, [b] see **Fig. 4**, [c] see **Fig. 8**. (*Reproduced from* Wieseler KM, Bhargava P, Kanal KM, et al. Imaging in pregnant patients: examination appropriateness. Radiographics 2010;30:1215–9; with permission.)

obstruction. Renal enlargement and perirenal fluid are suggestive of obstruction and absent in physiologic dilatation. In addition, physiologic dilatation shows a characteristic tapering because of extrinsic obstruction of the middle third of the ureter by the uterus.[11,53,54]

Low-dose CT can be performed if there is a high suspicion for lower tract calculi because CT has a higher sensitivity than US (**Fig. 7**).[45,46] CT also allows for the identification of alternative causes of flank pain.[3,11,25,36] The current trend of using low-dose multidetector CT coupled with the high accuracy (>95% sensitivity and >98% specificity) for the detection of calculi in the general population has lowered the threshold for the use of this technique as a second-line test in pregnancy. CT is now increasing being used in many institutions including that of the author. The algorithm used at the author's institution for imaging pregnant patients suspected of having urolithiasis is shown in **Fig. 8**.

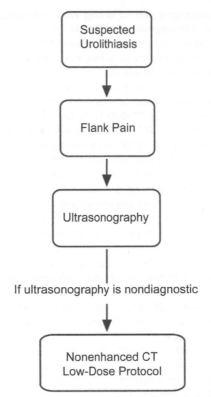

Fig. 8. Algorithm for workup of suspected urolithiasis in a pregnant patient. (*Reproduced from* Wieseler KM, Bhargava P, Kanal KM, et al. Imaging in pregnant patients: examination appropriateness. Radiographics 2010;30:1215–9; with permission.)

SUMMARY

In a pregnant patient, imaging is best performed using modalities that do not expose the fetus to ionizing radiation, such as US and MR imaging. Exposure to ionizing radiation can often be unavoidable, and, in such instances, the radiologist should develop an imaging plan in close consultation with the clinical team to obtain the diagnosis with the use of a single imaging diagnosis, with minimal delay. All efforts must be made by the radiologist to act as a guide both for the clinical team and the patient to minimize the fetal exposure and counsel the patient for radiation-associated risks. Risk versus benefit should be carefully assessed for a given scenario, and no imaging study should be withheld or deferred if an important clinical diagnosis is under consideration.

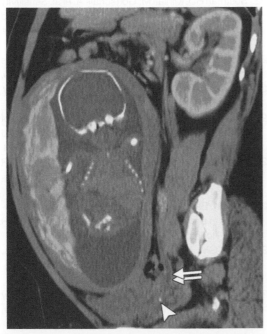

Fig. 7. Ureterovesical junction calculus in a 24-year-old patient in the second trimester with a history of left flank pain and hematuria. Urinalysis results were negative for infection except for hematuria. US performed earlier at another institution showed mild left hydronephrosis. CT was performed to investigate the cause of the hematuria. Oblique thick-section maximum-intensity-projection CT image shows the calculus (*arrowhead*) at the left ureterovesical junction with mild left hydroureter (*arrows*). (*Reproduced from* Wieseler KM, Bhargava P, Kanal KM, et al. Imaging in pregnant patients: examination appropriateness. Radiographics 2010;30:1215–9; with permission.)

REFERENCES

1. Ratnapalan S, Bona N, Chandra K, et al. Physicians' perceptions of teratogenic risk associated with

radiography and CT during early pregnancy. AJR Am J Roentgenol 2004;182:1107–9.

2. El-Khoury GY, Madsen MT, Blake ME, et al. A new pregnancy policy for a new era. AJR Am J Roentgenol 2003;181:335–40.

3. Wieseler KM, Bhargava P, Kanal KM, et al. Imaging in pregnant patients: examination appropriateness. Radiographics 2010;30:1215–29.

4. Coakley FV, Glenn OA, Qayyum A, et al. Fetal MRI: a developing technique for the developing patient. AJR Am J Roentgenol 2004;182:243–52.

5. American College of Radiology. ACR practice guideline for imaging pregnant or potentially pregnant adolescents and women with ionizing radiation. Reston (VA): American College of Radiology; 2008.

6. Martin JN Jr, Ridgway LE 3rd, Connors JJ, et al. Angiographic arterial embolization and computed tomography-directed drainage for the management of hemorrhage and infection with abdominal pregnancy. Obstet Gynecol 1990;76:941–5.

7. Bushberg JT. The essential physics of medical imaging. 2nd edition. Philadelphia: Lippincott Williams & Wilkins; 2002.

8. Wagner LK, Lester RG, Saldana LR. Exposure of the pregnant patient to diagnostic radiations: a guide to medical management. 2nd edition. Madison (WI): Medical Physics; 1997.

9. Brent RL. Saving lives and changing family histories: appropriate counseling of pregnant women and men and women of reproductive age, concerning the risk of diagnostic radiation exposures during and before pregnancy. Am J Obstet Gynecol 2009; 200:4–24.

10. Chen MM, Coakley FV, Kaimal A, et al. Guidelines for computed tomography and magnetic resonance imaging use during pregnancy and lactation. Obstet Gynecol 2008;112:333–40.

11. Patel SJ, Reede DL, Katz DS, et al. Imaging the pregnant patient for nonobstetric conditions: algorithms and radiation dose considerations. Radiographics 2007;27:1705–22.

12. Shellock FG, Crues JV. MR procedures: biologic effects, safety, and patient care. Radiology 2004; 232:635–52.

13. Webb JA, Thomsen HS, Morcos SK. Members of Contrast Media Safety Committee of European Society of Urogenital Radiology (ESUR). The use of iodinated and gadolinium contrast media during pregnancy and lactation. Eur Radiol 2005;15: 1234–40.

14. Pahade JK, Litmanovich D, Pedrosa I, et al. Quality initiatives: imaging pregnant patients with suspected pulmonary embolism: what the radiologist needs to know. Radiographics 2009;29:639–54.

15. Winer-Muram HT, Boone JM, Brown HL, et al. Pulmonary embolism in pregnant patients: fetal radiation dose with helical CT. Radiology 2002;224:487–92.

16. Scarsbrook AF, Evans AL, Owen AR, et al. Diagnosis of suspected venous thromboembolic disease in pregnancy. Clin Radiol 2006;61:1–12.

17. Nijkeuter M, Ginsberg JS, Huisman MV. Diagnosis of deep vein thrombosis and pulmonary embolism in pregnancy: a systematic review. J Thromb Haemost 2006;4:496–500.

18. Doshi SK, Negus IS, Oduko JM. Fetal radiation dose from CT pulmonary angiography in late pregnancy: a phantom study. Br J Radiol 2008;81:653–8.

19. Gotway MB, Reddy GP. Pulmonary thromboembolic disease. In: Webb WR, Higgins CB, editors. Thoracic imaging: pulmonary and cardiovascular radiology. 2nd edition. Philadelphia: Lippincott Williams & Wilkins; 2010.

20. Huda W, Slone R. Review of radiologic physics. 3rd edition. Philadelphia: Lippincott Williams & Wilkins; 2009.

21. Parker MS, Hui FK, Camacho MA, et al. Female breast radiation exposure during CT pulmonary angiography. AJR Am J Roentgenol 2005;185: 1228–33.

22. Sostman HD, Miniati M, Gottschalk A, et al. Sensitivity and specificity of perfusion scintigraphy combined with chest radiography for acute pulmonary embolism in PIOPED II. J Nucl Med 2008;49:1741–8.

23. Tamir IL, Bongard FS, Klein SR. Acute appendicitis in the pregnant patient. Am J Surg 1990;160:571–5.

24. Tracey M, Fletcher HS. Appendicitis in pregnancy. Am Surg 2000;66:555–9.

25. Pedrosa I, Zeikus EA, Levine D, et al. MR imaging of acute right lower quadrant pain in pregnant and nonpregnant patients. Radiographics 2007;27:721–43.

26. Pedrosa I, Levine D, Eyvazzadeh AD, et al. MR imaging evaluation of acute appendicitis in pregnancy. Radiology 2006;238:891–9.

27. Lim HK, Bae SH, Seo GS. Diagnosis of acute appendicitis in pregnant women: value of sonography. AJR Am J Roentgenol 1992;159:539–42.

28. Israel GM, Malguria N, McCarthy S, et al. MRI vs. ultrasound for suspected appendicitis during pregnancy. J Magn Reson Imaging 2008;28:428–33.

29. Cobben LP, Groot I, Haans L, et al. MRI for clinically suspected appendicitis during pregnancy. AJR Am J Roentgenol 2004;183:671–5.

30. Stone MB, Chao J. Emergency ultrasound diagnosis of acute appendicitis. Acad Emerg Med 2010;17:E5.

31. Kennedy A. Assessment of acute abdominal pain in the pregnant patient. Semin Ultrasound CT MR 2000;21:64–77.

32. Birchard KR, Brown MA, Hyslop WB, et al. MRI of acute abdominal and pelvic pain in pregnant patients. AJR Am J Roentgenol 2005;184:452–8.

33. Oto A, Ernst RD, Shah R, et al. Right-lower-quadrant pain and suspected appendicitis in pregnant women: evaluation with MR imaging–initial experience. Radiology 2005;234:445–51.

34. Vu L, Ambrose D, Vos P, et al. Evaluation of MRI for the diagnosis of appendicitis during pregnancy when ultrasound is inconclusive. J Surg Res 2009; 156:145–9.

35. Wagner LK, Huda W. When a pregnant woman with suspected appendicitis is referred for a CT scan, what should a radiologist do to minimize potential radiation risks? Pediatr Radiol 2004;34:589–90.

36. McCollough CH, Schueler BA, Atwell TD, et al. Radiation exposure and pregnancy: when should we be concerned? Radiographics 2007;27:909–17.

37. Maglinte DD, Bender GN, Heitkamp DE, et al. Multidetector-row helical CT enteroclysis. Radiol Clin North Am 2003;41:249–62.

38. Maglinte DD, Gourtsoyiannis N, Rex D, et al. Classification of small bowel Crohn's subtypes based on multimodality imaging. Radiol Clin North Am 2003; 41:285–303.

39. Lu EJ, Curet MJ, El-Sayed YY, et al. Medical versus surgical management of biliary tract disease in pregnancy. Am J Surg 2004;188:755–9.

40. Glasgow RE, Visser BC, Harris HW, et al. Changing management of gallstone disease during pregnancy. Surg Endosc 1998;12:241–6.

41. Shanmugam V, Beattie GC, Yule SR, et al. Is magnetic resonance cholangiopancreatography the new gold standard in biliary imaging? Br J Radiol 2005;78:888–93.

42. Moon JH, Cho YD, Cha SW, et al. The detection of bile duct stones in suspected biliary pancreatitis: comparison of MRCP, ERCP, and intraductal US. Am J Gastroenterol 2005;100:1051–7.

43. McAleer SJ, Loughlin KR. Nephrolithiasis and pregnancy. Curr Opin Urol 2004;14:123–7.

44. Parulkar BG, Hopkins TB, Wollin MR, et al. Renal colic during pregnancy: a case for conservative treatment. J Urol 1998;159:365–8.

45. Evans HJ, Wollin TA. The management of urinary calculi in pregnancy. Curr Opin Urol 2001;11: 379–84.

46. White WM, Zite NB, Gash J, et al. Low-dose computed tomography for the evaluation of flank pain in the pregnant population. J Endourol 2007; 21:1255–60.

47. Stothers L, Lee LM. Renal colic in pregnancy. J Urol 1992;148:1383–7.

48. Deyoe LA, Cronan JJ, Breslaw BH, et al. New techniques of ultrasound and color Doppler in the prospective evaluation of acute renal obstruction. Do they replace the intravenous urogram? Abdom Imaging 1995;20:58–63.

49. Wachsberg RH. Unilateral absence of ureteral jets in the third trimester of pregnancy: pitfall in color Doppler US diagnosis of urinary obstruction. Radiology 1998;209:279–81.

50. Hertzberg BS, Carroll BA, Bowie JD, et al. Doppler US assessment of maternal kidneys: analysis of intrarenal resistivity indexes in normal pregnancy and physiologic pelvicaliectasis. Radiology 1993; 186:689–92.

51. Shokeir AA, Mahran MR, Abdulmaaboud M. Renal colic in pregnant women: role of renal resistive index. Urology 2000;55:344–7.

52. Laing FC, Benson CB, DiSalvo DN, et al. Distal ureteral calculi: detection with vaginal US. Radiology 1994;192:545–8.

53. Roy C, Saussine C, LeBras Y, et al. Assessment of painful ureterohydronephrosis during pregnancy by MR urography. Eur Radiol 1996;6:334–8.

54. Spencer JA, Chahal R, Kelly A, et al. Evaluation of painful hydronephrosis in pregnancy: magnetic resonance urographic patterns in physiological dilatation versus calculous obstruction. J Urol 2004;171: 256–60.

Imaging the Pregnant Trauma Patient

Claudia Sadro, MD[a],*, Michelle Bittle, MD[a],
Kathy O'Connell, MN, RN[b]

KEYWORDS

- Trauma • Pregnant • Placental abruption
- External fetal monitoring

Trauma is the leading cause of nonobstetric maternal mortality[1] and affects approximately 7% of pregnancies.[2]

The most common causes of trauma in pregnancy are motor vehicle crashes and domestic violence. Other causes include different forms of assault or falls. Substance abuse may be a factor. Both major and minor traumas in pregnancy are associated with an increased risk of fetal loss.[3] The fetal loss rate due to blunt trauma ranges from 3.4% to 38.0%.[4] Most serious injuries result from motor vehicle crashes. Most pregnancy-related injuries occur in the third trimester of pregnancy.

Maternal death almost always results in fetal death. In rare third-trimester pregnancies, the fetus may be delivered by emergency cesarean delivery despite fatal maternal injuries, but this is the exception rather than the rule. The best chance for fetal survival is maternal survival, and all efforts are made to save the mother.[5]

TRAUMATIC INJURIES IN PREGNANCY

In major trauma, such as high-speed motor vehicle crashes frequently seen at level I trauma centers, the pregnant trauma patient is at risk for maternal injuries and uterine injuries. Maternal injuries include the same spectrum of injuries seen in nonpregnant trauma patients, such as injuries to the head, chest, abdomen, pelvis, vertebra, and extremities. Pregnant trauma patients are predisposed to certain types of injuries because of the physiologic changes of pregnancy. For example,

the blood volume increases 30% to 50% and uterine blood flow increases from 2% to 20% of the cardiac output.[4,6] There is enlargement of the ovarian veins making them prone to hemorrhage. The spleen enlarges increasing the risk of injury. The kidneys enlarge from hydronephrosis of pregnancy and are thus prone to injury. Uterine injuries include placental abruption, uterine laceration, and uterine rupture.[5] Fetal injuries are rare and are most commonly head injuries encountered in late third-trimester pregnancies in the setting of a maternal pelvic fracture.[4]

MANAGEMENT OF THE PREGNANT TRAUMA PATIENT

When the pregnant trauma patient presents to the emergency personnel, the ABC's are followed and the patient is resuscitated similar to any trauma patient, with additional considerations specific to the pregnancy. If the patient is more than 20 weeks pregnant, she is placed in the 30° left lateral decubitus position to prevent systemic hypotension caused by compression of the inferior vena cava by the gravid uterus.[7] Blood products are administered to maintain a hematocrit greater than 30% to optimize fetal oxygenation.[8] When the mother is stabilized, emergency ultrasonography is performed to determine the gestational age of the pregnancy and to determine if the fetus has a positive heart rate. Depending on the medical institution, the fetus is considered viable after 24 to 26 weeks of gestation or at a weight of 500 g.[4,5] For this and later gestational ages, the fetus is

[a] Harborview Medical Center, Department of Radiology, 325 Ninth Avenue, Seattle, WA 98104, USA
[b] Department of Obstetrics and Gynecology, University of Washington Medical Center, 1959 NE Pacific Street, Seattle, WA 98195, USA
* Corresponding author.
E-mail address: csadro@u.washington.edu

Ultrasound Clin 6 (2011) 97–103
doi:10.1016/j.cult.2010.11.002
1556-858X/11/$ – see front matter. Published by Elsevier Inc.

monitored continuously with external fetal monitoring. For gestational ages earlier than 24 to 28 weeks, the fetus is monitored intermittently because the fetus would not survive ex utero.

IMAGING THE PREGNANT TRAUMA PATIENT

In the setting of major trauma, the primary imaging modalities to evaluate for maternal injuries are radiography and computed tomography (CT). The role of ultrasonography is limited to fast scans to evaluate for free intraperitoneal fluid in unstable trauma patients in place of or as an adjunct to diagnostic peritoneal lavage and also to evaluate for pericardial fluid. Ultrasonography is used to evaluate fetal viability by identifying a fetal heart rate and determining the gestational age of the pregnancy. MR imaging is not practical in the acute trauma setting because it removes the patient from the direct care of emergency personnel and is time consuming. The seriously injured trauma patient may require angiography. CT, radiography, and fluoroscopy for angiography use ionizing radiation, and a fetus is more susceptible to the harmful effects of ionizing radiation than children and adults. However, in the setting of major trauma, the risks of ionizing radiation to the fetus from these imaging studies are minimal compared to the risks of not diagnosing trauma to the mother in a timely fashion, and these imaging studies are performed without delay. This practice is supported by the American College of Radiology. Pregnant trauma patients are imaged in the same manner as nonpregnant trauma patients. Intravenous iodinated contrast is a Food and Drug Administration class B agent and is given in pregnancy in the trauma setting. Very little intravenous iodinated contrast crosses the placenta into the fetal circulation, and there are no known adverse effects to the fetus.[9]

RADIATION AND PREGNANCY

The American College of Obstetricians and Gynecologists Committee Opinion on Guidelines for Diagnostic Imaging in Pregnancy from 2004 states "Women should be counseled that x ray exposure from a single diagnostic procedure does not result in harmful fetal effects. Specifically, exposure to less than 5 rad (50 mGy) has not been associated with an increase in fetal anomalies or pregnancy loss."[10] This opinion is also supported by the National Council on Radiation Protection and Measurements Report No 54 from 1977 that states "The risk (of abnormality) is considered to be negligible at 5 rad (50 mGy) or less when compared to the other risks of pregnancy, and the risk of

malformations is significantly increased above control levels only at doses above 15 rad (150 mGy)."[11]

Radiation dose is measured in the rad (radiation absorbed dose) and the rem (radiation equivalent in man). In the International System of units, the rad is expressed as the Gray and the rem as the Sievert. For diagnostic imaging that uses low-energy radiation in the form of x-rays and γ rays, 1 rad = 1 rem = 10 mGy = 10 mSv.[12] **Table 1** shows the typical fetal doses in millisieverts for common radiological procedures and compares them to the background radiation dose to the fetus for 9 months of pregnancy. The background radiation dose to the fetus for 9 months of pregnancy is 0.5 to 1.0 mSv.[5,13] Radiography and CT scans in which the fetus is not in the field of view result in a very low fetal radiation dose, less than or similar to the background dose. Examinations that have the fetus in the field of view result in a relatively high fetal radiation dose. The typical fetal dose for a CT abdomen/pelvis is 25 mSv. In trauma, a CT lumbar spine and CT bony pelvis can be reconstructed from the CT abdomen/pelvis so that the fetus is only irradiated once. In serious trauma, in which there is concern for renal or bladder injury or active contrast extravasation,

Table 1
Typical fetal radiation doses for common radiological procedures compared to the background fetal radiation dose for 9 months of pregnancy

Examination	Typical Fetal Dose (mGy)
Cervical spine (AP, lat) or extremities	<0.001[13]
Chest radiography (PA, lat)	<0.002[13]
Abdomen (AP)	21 cm patient thickness 1 33 cm patient thickness 3[13]
Lumbar spine (AP, lat)	1[13]
CT head	0[13]
CT chest or CTPA	0.2[13]
CT abdomen/pelvis	25[13]
Fluoroscopy	20–100 mGy/min[5]
Background radiation for 9 months of pregnancy	0.5–1.0[13]

1 rad = 1 rem = 10 mGy = 10 mSv.
Abbreviations: AP, anteroposterior; CTPA, CT pulmonary angiography; lat, lateral; PA, posteroanterior.

a second pass lower-dose delayed scan may be necessary. If there is concern for active bleeding, angiography may be performed for identification and embolization of bleeding vessels. The fetal radiation dose for fluoroscopy when the fetus is in the field of view is 20 to 100 mGy/min, depending on the number of spot films obtained.[5]

The risk of ionizing radiation to the fetus depends on the gestational age and fetal radiation dose.[14] Less than 2 weeks postconception, the main risk of ionizing radiation to the fetus is spontaneous abortion. It is an all-or-none response. After 15 weeks post conception, the main risk of ionizing radiation to pregnancy is childhood cancer, mainly childhood leukemia. The baseline risk of fatal childhood cancer is 0.05%, and the relative risk after exposure to 50 mGy is 2. The odds of dying from childhood cancer range from 1 per 2000 (baseline) to 2 per 2000 after an exposure of 50 mGy, which is still very low.[9] Less than 2 weeks postconception and after 15 weeks post conception, regardless of the radiation dose to the fetus, therapeutic abortion is not recommended during patient counseling. The only stage of pregnancy when exposure of the fetus to ionizing radiation may be sufficiently high to discuss therapeutic abortion with the mother is the period of organogenesis between 2 and 15 weeks postconception. Between 2 and 15 weeks postconception, the risks of ionizing radiation to the pregnancy are small head size, mental retardation, organ malformations, and childhood cancer. The first 3 risks are absent when the fetal radiation dose is less than 50 mSv and are low when the dose is less than 100 mSv. Therefore, therapeutic abortion is not typically recommended until the fetal radiation dose exceeds 150 mSv during this stage of pregnancy.[14]

Unless the mother is seriously injured, requiring multiple imaging examinations, the fetal radiation dose from diagnostic imaging procedures performed in trauma rarely exceeds 50 mSv. Rarely, the fetal radiation dose approaches 100 or 150 mSv, and the fetus survives the trauma. The pregnant trauma patient is imaged in the same manner as a nonpregnant trauma patient. Informed consent is not obtained in seriously injured patients. A thermoluminescent dosimeter is placed on the abdomen of the pregnant patient, and the skin entrance dose is calculated. If the skin entrance dose exceeds a certain threshold determined by an individual institution, a physicist should perform a detailed dose calculation. After the dose calculation, an addendum is included in the patient's radiology report that includes an estimation of the dose of radiation exposure to the fetus and the risk category. The mother should be counseled in hospital about the radiation exposure to the fetus and the risks.

EXAMPLES OF TRAUMATIC INJURIES SPECIFIC TO THE PREGNANT TRAUMA PATIENT
Placental Abruption

In cases of trauma when the mother survives, the most common cause of fetal death is placental abruption. Placental abruption occurs with both major and minor traumas.[15] It is most common after 16 weeks gestation.[4] The placenta is more rigid than the more compliant uterine wall. With trauma, shearing forces occur between the placenta and the uterine wall resulting in hemorrhage and uteroplacental separation (**Fig. 1**). Subchorionic abruption, that occurs between the placenta and uterine wall, includes marginal and retroplacental abruption. Marginal abruption occurs between the peripheral margin of the placenta and the uterine wall. Retroplacental abruption occurs more centrally between the placenta and uterine wall and has a worse prognosis. When more than 30% to 40% of the surface area of the placenta is involved, placental abruption is severe and is associated with a 50% fetal mortality.[8] Preplacental or subamniotic abruption may also occur but is of no clinical significance.

The diagnosis of placental abruption may be suspected clinically. Patients typically present with uterine pain and vaginal bleeding. Approximately 80% of patients with placental abruption have vaginal bleeding, and the blood is maternal blood. Approximately 20% of patients with placental abruption have a concealed abruption without vaginal bleeding. With more advanced placental abruption, patients have increased uterine tone and fetal heart rate abnormalities. The most sensitive test to diagnose placental abruption is external fetal monitoring with devices that measure uterine contractility and fetal heart rate.[8] All pregnant trauma patients who are more than 24 weeks pregnant should be monitored with continuous external fetal monitoring for at least 4 hours after their trauma.[15] Signs of placental abruption are increased uterine contractions, increased uterine tone, fetal heart rate decelerations, and bradycardia. Abnormalities in the fetal heart rate tracing including late decelerations and a bradycardia of less than 80 beats per minute indicate fetal distress and hypoxemia that warrant emergency cesarean delivery.[8] **Fig. 2** shows the external fetal monitoring of a pregnant patient who has severe placental abruption warranting emergency cesarean delivery.

Ultrasonography is often requested to diagnose placental abruption. Unfortunately, ultrasonography

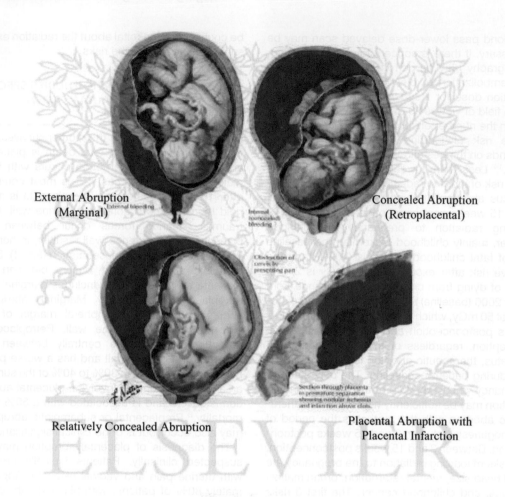

External Abruption (Marginal)

Concealed Abruption (Retroplacental)

Relatively Concealed Abruption

Placental Abruption with Placental Infarction

Fig. 1. Placental abruption (or premature separation of the placenta). Subchorionic: marginal abruption and retroplacental abruption. (*Reprinted from* Netter Anatomy Illustration Collection, © Elsevier Inc. All Rights Reserved.)

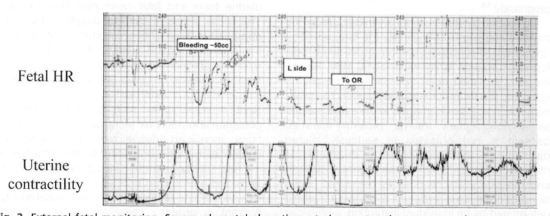

Fetal HR

Uterine contractility

Fig. 2. External fetal monitoring. Severe placental abruption: uterine contractions are occurring every minute with increasing baseline tone as the tracing evolves. The fetal heart rate demonstrates a variable-appearing deceleration evolving into a prolonged fetal deceleration. Toward the end of the tracing, the fetal heart rate is lost entirely. When it returns there is fetal bradycardia measuring 70 to 80 beats per minute, indicating fetal distress and hypoxemia. The patient had an emergency cesarean delivery. L, left; HR, heart rate; OR, operating room. (*Courtesy of* Kathy O'Connell, MN, RN, University of Washington Medical Center, Seattle, WA.)

is insensitive and gives false-negative results in 50% to 80% of cases. Nonetheless, there are some sonographic signs that suggest the diagnosis of placental abruption. **Fig. 3** shows ultrasonographic results on a pregnant trauma patient, demonstrating placental abruption. Early on, focal enlargement of the placenta with retroplacental clot is observed. The retroplacental clot may be isoechoic to placenta in which case the placenta just appears focally enlarged. Alternatively, it may be hyperechoic, hypoechoic, or of mixed echogenicity (see **Fig. 3**A). It can be distinguished from the normal retroplacental venous plexus by the lack of blood flow on color Doppler imaging. Over time, a resolving retroplacental clot becomes hypoechoic and decreases in size (see **Fig. 3**B). Other signs include echogenic amniotic fluid because of bleeding into the amniotic cavity and echogenic fetal bowel because of the fetus swallowing the blood.[16]

The diagnosis of placental abruption can also be made on contrast-enhanced CT.[17] Contrast enhanced CT is not performed specifically to diagnose placental abruption. However, if a pregnant patient is involved in trauma that is serious enough to warrant investigation with CT to evaluate for maternal injuries, the diagnosis of placental abruption can be made by CT. On CT, placental abruption results in focal enlargement of the placenta with diminished enhancement at the site of the retroplacental clot. There may be placental infarction with diminished enhancement extending from the placental base to the placental surface (**Fig. 4**). In more serious cases, hyperdense amniotic fluid may be present because of bleeding into the amniotic cavity.

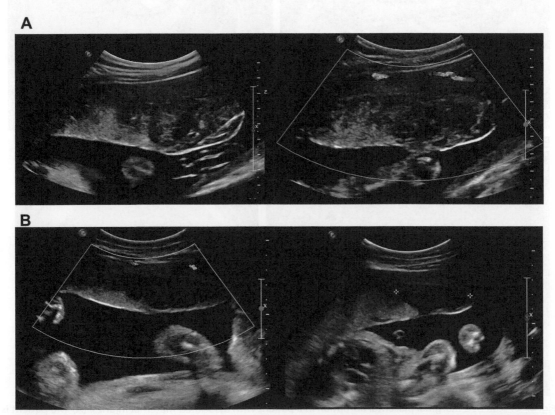

Fig. 3. Ultrasonography of retroplacental abruption posttrauma. (*A*) Patient is a 19-year-old female and is 24 weeks pregnant. She sustained blunt trauma to the abdomen 1 week prior in a mosh pit. She received multiple blows to the abdomen (moshing is a form of slam dancing at music concerts). She had uterine contractions over the past week. The day before admission and performing ultrasonography, she had severe abdominal pain and vaginal bleeding. Ultrasonography shows thickening of the placenta with clot of heterogeneous echogenicity between the placenta and uterine wall without internal flow to color Doppler assessment. The size of the clot measured 3.5 × 10 × 10 cm. (*B*) A follow-up ultrasonography performed 3 weeks later shows an interval decrease in size of the retroplacental clot that has become hypoechoic over time without internal color flow. The clot now measures 2.3 × 4.8 × 9.3 cm. The patient did not have premature rupture of membranes, and the vaginal bleeding and uterine contractions had stopped. She was discharged home with arrangements made for close interval follow-up.

Risk factors for placental abruption, other than trauma, include low socioeconomic status, multiparity, history of placental abruption, retroplacental fibroids, cocaine or tobacco use, maternal hypertension, maternal coagulopathy, and chorioamnionitis. Complications of placental abruption include fetal death, preterm labor, maternal coagulopathy, intrauterine growth retardation, and oligohydramnios.[8]

Uterine Laceration and Uterine Rupture

Other complications of trauma in pregnancy are uterine laceration and uterine rupture. Uterine rupture may result from trauma, particularly in patients who have had a prior cesarean delivery. It occurs following major trauma, and the fetal death rate approaches 100%. Imaging features include a free floating fetus, free intraperitoneal

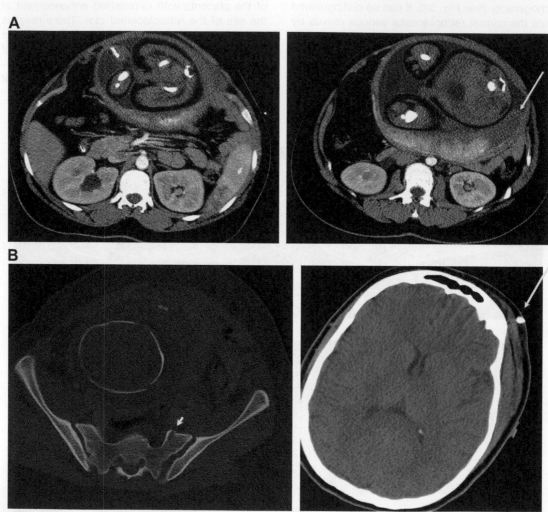

Fig. 4. CT scan of a marginal placental abruption in a patient with associated maternal injuries. (*A*) The patient is 34 weeks pregnant and was involved in a T-bone motor vehicle crash. The patient was a restrained driver and collided with a tractor trailer while making a left turn at 35 mph. The patient was intubated in the field. CT of the abdomen and pelvis with intravenous contrast shows a grade 2 splenic laceration (*short arrow*) and marginal placental abruption with infarction (*long arrow*). There is diminished enhancement in the left side of the placenta, extending from the placental base to the placental surface. Maternal hydronephrosis of pregnancy can be noticed on the right. (*B*) The patient sustained a pelvic fracture (*short arrow*) and a head injury with glass embedded in the scalp in the left frontal region (*long arrow*). A limited obstetric ultrasonography showed normal results. She had external fetal monitoring that initially showed irregular uterine contractions. She then developed painful uterine contractions and nonreactive fetal heart tracings. She was diagnosed with severe placental abruption and underwent emergency cesarean delivery. She also had a splenorrhaphy and delivered a normal infant.

fluid representing amniotic fluid and blood, and an empty uterine cavity.[6,18]

SUMMARY

Trauma is the leading cause of nonobstetric maternal mortality. Maternal death usually results in fetal death, and the best chance for fetal survival is maternal survival. When the mother survives, the most common cause of fetal death is placental abruption. Fetal loss occurs with both major and minor traumas. All pregnant trauma patients must be monitored closely. In high-energy trauma, such as motor vehicle crashes, the pregnant trauma patient is imaged in the same way as a nonpregnant trauma patient, with radiography, CT, and angiography, as needed. Ultrasonography is limited to fast scans in unstable patients and to evaluate the viability of the pregnancy. The risks of ionizing radiation to the fetus are minimal when compared to the risks of trauma to the mother and her pregnancy. The radiation exposure to the fetus from diagnostic imaging in trauma almost never warrants termination of the pregnancy. The risks are discussed with the mother during her hospital stay. In low-energy trauma when there is no concern for maternal injuries but there is concern for placental abruption, the patient undergoes external fetal monitoring and ultrasonography of the gravid uterus. Ultrasonography is insensitive in diagnosing placental abruption and shows false-negative results in 50% to 80% of cases. The most sensitive approach for diagnosing placental abruption is external fetal monitoring. Abnormal fetal heart tones are an indication for emergency cesarean delivery in cases of suspected placental abruption.

REFERENCES

1. Fildes J, Reed L, Jones N, et al. Trauma: the leading cause of maternal death. J Trauma 1992; 32(5):643–5.
2. Towery R, English TP, Wisner D, et al. Evaluation of pregnant women after blunt injury. J Trauma 1993; 35(5):731–5 [discussion: 735–6].
3. Mattox KL, Goetzl L. Trauma in pregnancy. Crit Care Med 2005;33(Suppl 10):S385–9.
4. Grossman NB. Blunt trauma in pregnancy. Am Fam Physician 2004;70(7):1303–10.
5. Bernstein MP. Imaging of traumatic injuries in pregnancy. State of the Art Emergency and Trauma Radiology. American Roentgen Ray Society Course and Syllabus 2008:203–10.
6. Goldman SM, Wagner LK. Radiologic management of abdominal trauma in pregnancy. AJR Am J Roentgenol 1996;166(4):763–7.
7. Milsom I, Forssman L. Factors influencing aortocaval compression in late pregnancy. Am J Obstet Gynecol 1984;148(6):764–71.
8. Kay HH. Danforth's obstetrics and gynecology. Lippincott Williams & Wilkins; 2008.
9. Chen MM, Coakley FV, Kaimal A, et al. Guidelines for computed tomography and magnetic resonance imaging use during pregnancy and lactation. Obstet Gynecol 2008;112(2 Pt 1):333–40.
10. ACOG Committee on Obstetric Practice. ACOG Committee Opinion. Number 299, September 2004 (replaces No. 158, September 1995). Guidelines for diagnostic imaging during pregnancy. Obstet Gynecol 2004;104(3):647–51.
11. Medical radiation exposure of pregnant and potentially pregnant women: National Council on Radiation Protection and Measurements Report No 54.
12. Huda W. Review of radiologic physics. 3rd edition. Philadelphia (PA): Wolters Kluwer. Lippincott Williams and Wilkins; 2010.
13. McCollough CH, Schueler BA, Atwell TD, et al. Radiation exposure and pregnancy: when should we be concerned? Radiographics 2007;27(4):909–17 [discussion: 917–8].
14. Wagner L. Exposure of the pregnant patient to diagnostic radiations. Madison (WI): Medical Physics Publishing; 1997.
15. Pearlman MD, Tintinalli JE, Lorenz RP. Blunt trauma during pregnancy. N Engl J Med 1990;323(23): 1609–13.
16. STATdx Diagnostic Imaging for Radiologists. eBook. Salt Lake City (UT): Amirsys, Inc; 2005–2010.
17. Wei SH, Helmy M, Cohen AJ, et al. CT evaluation of placental abruption in pregnant trauma patients. Emerg Radiol 2009;16(5):365–73.
18. Harrison SD, Nghiem HV, Shy K, et al. Uterine rupture with fetal death following blunt trauma. AJR Am J Roentgenol 1995;165(6):1452.

Fetal and Perinatal Death Investigation: Redefining the Autopsy and the Role of Radiologic Imaging

Corinne L. Fligner, MD[a],*, Manjiri Dighe, MD[b]

KEYWORDS

- Autopsy • Postmortem • Imaging • Radiology
- MRI • Fetal • Minimally invasive

Autopsy is the examination of a body after death, and traditionally has been viewed as a procedure performed by pathologists using dissection. However, autopsy is more correctly viewed as the final opportunity for the examination of a (deceased) individual, with the goal of diagnosing disease and in some cases determining the cause of death. Traditionally, the autopsy performed by the pathologist includes an external examination of the body, internal examination with dissection, photographic documentation of external and internal features, and histologic evaluation. Fetal autopsy may allow delineation of anomalies, establishment of an etiology for abnormalities, determination of cause of death or intrauterine demise, and correlation of pathologic features with antemortem radiologic and other diagnostic studies for quality-assurance purposes. Autopsy diagnoses can assist families and clinicians in understanding the cause of fetal abnormalities or problems in the pregnancy, as well as providing objective information about prognosis in future pregnancies, to assist with both counseling and management of a future pregnancy.

Advances in prenatal ultrasound and magnetic resonance (MR) imaging have prompted increased interest in the use of these imaging techniques in the postmortem setting to augment or substitute for a traditional autopsy examination. In recent years, there has been a continued decrease in the percentage of fetal and infant autopsies. Reasons cited for this decline include absence of reimbursement for autopsy, lack of interest by pathologists, and lack of pathologist expertise. In addition, increasingly diverse populations have resulted in more families in which traditional pathologic dissection is precluded by cultural or religious beliefs.[1] More recently, the widely publicized investigations in the United Kingdom into retention of organs and tissues without family permission have had considerable effect on the negative view of fetal and infant autopsy by families.[1–3] A governmental mandate with associated funding has resulted in a body of research in the United Kingdom focused on the development and validation of noninvasive, radiologic imaging techniques to investigate fetal and infant deaths without the use of traditional autopsy dissection, with a goal of identifying noninvasive

---

The authors have nothing to disclose.

[a] Anatomic Pathology–Autopsy and After Death Services, Division of Anatomic Pathology, University of Washington Medical Center (UWMC), Departments of Pathology and Laboratory Medicine, University of Washington School of Medicine, Box 356100, Seattle, WA 98195, USA

[b] Radiology–Body Imaging, University of Washington Medical Center (UWMC), Department of Radiology, University of Washington School of Medicine, Box 357115, Seattle, WA 98195, USA

* Corresponding author.

E-mail address: fligner@u.washington.edu

Ultrasound Clin 6 (2011) 105–117

doi:10.1016/j.cult.2011.01.003

imaging procedures that could be equivalent to traditional autopsy in many circumstances.[2–10]

This article describes some of the major features of the conventional or traditional fetal/infant autopsy, discusses the current research in postmortem radiologic imaging, including advantages and limitations, and suggests an approach for the integrative use of multiple specialized examinations in the investigation of fetal and infant deaths.

THE FETAL AUTOPSY: PATHOLOGY
Administrative Issues

In the United States, autopsies are performed in 2 general settings: medical-legal autopsies do not require the consent of the legal next of kin, and medical or hospital autopsies cannot be performed without consent from the legal next of kin. Although the statutory requirements for medical-legal autopsies vary by location or jurisdiction, the focus of the coroner and medical examiner systems in which these autopsies are performed is the investigation of sudden and unexpected, apparently natural deaths, and deaths related to injury of many types. Perinatal and fetal deaths that would likely be investigated and autopsied in the medical-legal system could include the unexpected death of a neonate or infant, including those ultimately classified as being caused by sudden infant death syndrome; some pregnancy-related deaths of the mother and/or fetus/infant; fetal/perinatal deaths caused by maternal injury of any type (eg, a motor-vehicle collision, or inflicted injury of the mother); fetal death caused by possible illegal abortion; and fetal and/or infant death related to inflicted injury or neglect and, in some settings, caused by maternal drug use.

Most fetal and perinatal autopsies are performed in the hospital setting (so-called hospital or medical autopsies), and are performed only with consent of the legal next of kin, usually 1 or both parents. It is important that the autopsy consent is sufficiently explicit to allow families to make an informed decision about autopsy and what procedures are acceptable to them, with any nonstandard autopsy procedures requiring specific consent. The consenting family member can limit or restrict the autopsy procedure based on their wishes. In the medical setting, consent for autopsy is required for any formal examination or invasive procedure performed on the body after death, including those examinations that are not, or are only minimally, invasive, such as external examinations, radiologic evaluations, photography, and needle or skin biopsies.

In the United States autopsy consent was not always required for examination and dissection of a fetus younger than the gestational age at which a death certificate was required, this requirement varying by state. Each state requires a death certificate for a fetus older than a certain gestational age or weighing more than a specified weight. For example, in the state of Washington, a Fetal Death Certificate is required for any still-born fetus older than 20 weeks' gestation, and a regular death certificate is required for any live-born fetus or infant of any gestational age.[11] However, many institutions, including the University of Washington Medical Center, require autopsy consent for an examination to be performed on any intact fetus, no matter what the gestational age. This requirement ensures that the family understands and actively consents to the autopsy procedure, or limits the procedure based on counseling and their specific wishes.

Fetal and perinatal autopsies are ideally performed by a pathologist with expertise, interest, and experience in this subspecialty of pediatric pathology, often, but not always a board-certified pediatric pathologist.

Autopsy Procedure: Pathology

The autopsy examination begins with a review of the clinical history, prenatal laboratory studies, and radiologic images, and discussion of the clinical questions with the clinical provider and/or genetic counselor. Review of antenatal imaging may assist in determining whether postmortem imaging might be helpful, as in the setting of possible structural abnormalities of the brain. Early assessment of the need for tissue samples for cytogenetic or molecular diagnostic evaluation allows prompt and timely sampling to better ensure viable fibroblast cultures and well-preserved DNA samples.

The autopsy procedure for a fetus or infant has been described in detail in several publications.[12–14] The external examination is critically important, because it can exclude abnormalities as well as identify and etiologically clarify observed anomalies. The external examination includes standard measurements such as weight, foot length, crown-rump and crown-heel lengths, and occipital-frontal circumference, which can be compared with charts of standard measurements for gestational age. Intraoral examination with attention to the pharynx and assessment of the soft palate and uvula allow evaluation for subtle degrees of cleft palate. Attention should be paid to joint mobility, facial features, and the appearance of the hands, feet, and external genitalia.

To prevent misdiagnosis, the pathologist should be familiar with the normal appearance of fetuses at different gestational ages, and the changes related to the postmortem autolysis (maceration) that occurs after intrauterine demise.

Photographic documentation of external features is critical, because photographs can be reviewed by other experts, especially geneticists, correlated with antemortem imaging, and archived for future review in evaluation of a possible recurrence in a subsequent pregnancy. Use of a digital camera with a macroscopic lens optimizes documentation of early gestation fetuses. Some photographs should include a scale and identifying number, and the subject and background should be free of blood or other distracting objects such as towels or sponges. Standard photographs should generally include an overall photograph of the anterior body, and anterior and lateral views of the face. All external abnormalities should be photographed, particularly those involving the face, ears, extremities, and genitalia; photographs to illustrate pertinent negatives may be useful.

The internal examination of the chest and abdomen is usually associated with a Y- or T-shaped incision on the anterior trunk. Organs are examined in situ in detail, with particular attention to anatomic position and configuration, and the delineation of the vascular connections of the heart. In many cases, the heart is opened in situ, and the organs are usually removed en bloc for detailed dissection (Rokitansky method). Common modifications to the standard dissection procedure may include removal and fixation of the heart and lungs before dissection, when there is concern about structural cardiac abnormalities, and fixation of the organ bloc before dissection in the presence of marked autolysis, for improved anatomic detail. The spinal cord can be easily removed by an internal anterior approach, by removing the anterior vertebral column and unroofing the spinal canal.

Removal of the brain is usually accomplished by use of a coronal scalp incision extending to behind the ears, with the otherwise intact scalp reflected anteriorly and posteriorly along the incision. The skull is opened by cutting along the cranial sutures, opening the calvarial skull and examining the cerebrum first. When there is antenatal suspicion of intracranial posterior fossa abnormalities, such as Dandy-Walker malformation complex or Chiari malformation, better visualization of posterior fossa abnormalities is achieved by using a posterior approach to extend the coronal scalp incision into the posterior neck region. After removal of the occipital bone and the posterior cervical vertebral elements (**Fig. 1**), the posterior fossa is visualized before evaluation of the supratentorial structures by incision along the sutures.

The fetal and infant brain is extremely soft, because of high water content, and is best examined internally by dissection after about a week to 10 days of fixation in 10% buffered formalin. Increased firmness of the brain improves internal evaluation, and can be achieved by adding a small amount of acetic acid to the formalin solution (Joseph R. Siebert, PhD, personal communication, 2010). In some cases, in situ injection of the cerebral ventricles with buffered formalin, followed by several days of fixation, may optimize the internal anatomic delineation. Even using these techniques, detailed evaluation of structural abnormalities is difficult because tissue fragility often results in structural disruption during removal, which is exacerbated in the setting of postmortem autolysis. Evaluation of the cranial base is important, particularly when the brain is autolyzed, because the identification of a normal configuration of the anterior cranial fossa with a normal crista galli and cribriform plate allows exclusion of alobar and semilobar holoprosencephaly.

During the internal examination, samples of normal and abnormal tissues are obtained for histologic evaluation. In addition, if cytogenetic studies or DNA preservation is requested, fresh tissue should be placed in tissue culture media. Because it is not always known whether specialized ancillary studies requiring frozen, unfixed tissue may be needed for diagnosis, it is useful to follow a standard protocol for the routine sampling and retention of tissue for possible additional ancillary studies, in which fetal liver and fetal surface of the placenta are separately frozen and retained in every case.[15,16] Additional tissue might be frozen on a case-by-case basis; for example, in a fetus with arthrogryposis, freezing skeletal muscle for detailed histochemistry might be indicated, depending on the condition of the body. For fetuses for which blood is available, a blood card can be obtained and retained indefinitely for subsequent DNA testing. For standard sampling for cytogenetics, a skin biopsy, including fascia and skeletal muscle, can be obtained from the lateral thigh, or from any area of relatively well-preserved skin. In addition, lung and kidney are also samples that are more likely to result in fibroblast growth for cytogenetic purposes, when skin samples do not. Amnion or superficial placenta obtained from the fetal surface of the placenta may also be a source of viable cells when there is autolysis of fetal tissues. When organs or tissues are used to directly prepare DNA for testing or retention, lung, kidney, skeletal muscle, gonad, and umbilical cord are good sources.

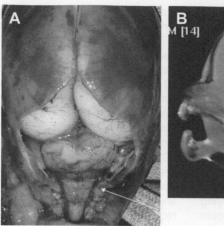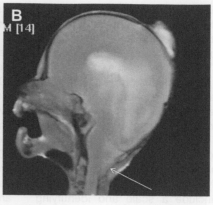

Fig. 1. (*A*) Chiari II malformation at autopsy shown by posterior approach for visualization of the posterior cranial fossa. Arrow located at the inferior aspect of posterior fossa, showing the inferior displacement of the medulla oblongata. (*B*) Postmortem T1-weighted MR image shows similar features of small posterior fossa and inferior displacement of the vermis (*arrow*) in another case of lumbosacral neural tube defect with Chiari II malformation.

Autopsy: Ancillary Studies

Several ancillary studies are important in the investigation of fetal and infant death. Macroscopic and microscopic examination of the placenta is a critical component of the fetal autopsy, particularly in the setting of intrauterine demise, fetal hydrops, and intrauterine growth restriction.[17] A recent review of 104 consecutive perinatal deaths (2005–2008), of gestational age ranging from 22 weeks to 7 days post partum, of which 78% were intrauterine fetal demise, showed that in 70% of the cases, placental changes could explain the fetal death, and in 48%, the death was explained by placental examination only. The placenta can also be an excellent source for tissue for cytogenetic studies or DNA extraction, and placental cytogenetics might be indicated in the setting of severe growth restriction concerning for confined placental mosaicism. Other ancillary studies include cytogenetic evaluations (karyotype, array comparative genomic hybridization); molecular (genetic) diagnostic studies; maternal laboratory studies such as infectious serologies, Kleihauer-Betke test for fetal maternal hemorrhage, and tests for autoantibodies or antiphospholipid antibodies or inherited coagulophilias; and microbiologic culture or molecular diagnostic studies of placental or fetal tissues to evaluate infectious causes.

Identification of an integrative diagnosis or a list of diagnostic possibilities requires correlation of pathologic findings with clinical, radiologic, and molecular diagnostic results, and close collaboration with clinical geneticists and genetic counselors. Several online resources are available to assist in this effort, including Online Mendelian Inheritance in Man (OMIM)[18] and GeneClinics[19]; the latter reference includes a dynamic list of laboratories performing testing in both research and clinical settings for many inherited diseases.

ROLE OF ANTENATAL IMAGING IN DEATH INVESTIGATION

Antenatal ultrasound imaging is the major modality for the detection of structural abnormalities of the fetus and placenta. The detection of abnormalities on ultrasound may prompt performance of imaging that can more specifically delineate those abnormalities, such as cranial MR imaging or fetal echocardiography, or three-dimensional image reconstruction to more clearly visualize facial anomalies such as cleft lip. Knowledge of the ultrasound abnormalities can allow the pathologist to modify the pathologic examination for optimal demonstration of findings, and in some instances, to examine regions and/or remove tissues for histologic examination that would not be examined in a routine autopsy.

Many studies have been performed to evaluate the diagnostic accuracy of ultrasound when compared with autopsy or pathologic examination after termination of pregnancy. For example, Akgun and colleagues[20] reported a 4-year-long prospective study of 107 second-trimester fetuses with malformations diagnosed by second-trimester ultrasound. All the major anomalies leading to termination of pregnancy were confirmed by fetal autopsy, with an overall success rate for detection of anomalies of 77%. The most frequent prenatally diagnosed malformations were in the central nervous system (CNS) (49%), with hydrocephalus and neural tube defects most common, followed by renal and cardiac abnormalities. In 20% of cases, additional minor findings were detected at autopsy. There were 4 cases in which the prenatally diagnosed CNS anomalies could not be identified because of autolysis.

Although ultrasound findings generally correlate well with pathologic findings, the sensitivity varies with the type of anomaly, with more limited sensitivity for some developmental and acquired (destructive) CNS anomalies. For example, Phillips and colleagues[21] noted that correlation between a prenatal ultrasound diagnosis of Dandy-Walker malformation complex and autopsy neuropathology findings were poor, with a 55% rate of concordance. These investigators' retrospective study of 44 cases suggested that an unequivocal ultrasonographic diagnosis of Dandy-Walker malformation complex be reserved for cases with the classic findings of Dandy-Walker malformation, including enlargement of the cisterna magna, aplasia of the vermis, and a trapezoid, rather than keyhole-shaped, interhemispheric gap, and they identified specific neuropathologic techniques to increase the diagnostic accuracy of this diagnosis. Likewise, some cases of cystic renal disease are notably difficult to specifically diagnose either by antemortem ultrasound or MR imaging (**Fig. 2**), and require pathologic evaluation of the kidney, both grossly and microscopically, with molecular diagnostic correlation, to determine the specific diagnosis.[22] Particularly in areas of rapid evolution, such as the characterization of fetal cystic renal disease, use of all modalities available for evaluation optimally allows specific diagnosis.

Antenatal MR imaging is now considered an important diagnostic modality in the evaluation of abnormalities of the fetal CNS, and is reported to detect abnormalities that are not identified by ultrasound in up to 50% of cases, and conversely, to show normal imaging findings in settings in which the ultrasound suggested abnormality. Abnormalities in which antenatal MR imaging using T2-weighted images can be particularly helpful include posterior fossa abnormalities such as Dandy-Walker malformation complex, arachnoid cysts, and cerebellar malformations; cortical developmental abnormalities, including lissencephaly, polymicrogyria, schizencephaly, and porencephaly; and congenital infections, such as cytomegalovirus. Dean and Whitby have described the complementary interaction of antenatal MR imaging and neuropathology, which allows

compensation for the difficulties of fetal neuropathology (eg, localization of small abnormal structures that cannot be identified macroscopically) and for the limitations of fetal MR imaging, including less detailed resolution, absence of etiologic specificity, and absence of histologic diagnosis.[23]

POSTMORTEM RADIOLOGIC IMAGING

In the last few decades, there has been increasing interest and research in the use of radiologic imaging other than plain radiographs in the postmortem setting. Many early studies of postmortem imaging were performed in the forensic setting, with efforts toward developing a virtual autopsy to allow in situ visualization of the effects of trauma not possible with the traditional autopsy. In the forensic evaluation of infant or child death, plain-film skeletal imaging has long been an important modality for showing and evaluating recent or healed bony fractures, and more recently, for showing intracranial injury.

Postmortem Imaging: Plain Radiographs and Computed Tomography Scans

Postmortem radiography of fetuses and infants is a critical component in the evaluation of skeletal dysplasia. Although prenatal ultrasound studies can identify abnormalities of bone formation and growth, specific diagnosis or exclusion of a skeletal dysplasia generally requires evaluation of plain radiographs.[24] In the evaluation of a skeletal dysplasia, the combination of plain-film radiography in conjunction with an external examination performed by a pathologist or geneticist and photographs of the fetus may often comprise a pathologic examination adequate for diagnosis. Ideally, radiographs should be reviewed by a pediatric radiologist with expertise in skeletal dysplasia. The films can confirm some diagnoses not identifiable by ultrasound, such as thanatophoric dysplasia or achondrogenesis type 1B, as well as identify features such as chondrodysplasia punctata, which can direct additional molecular diagnostic and/or biochemical studies (**Figs. 3 and 4**). Identification of fractures can direct studies toward disorders of collagen synthesis, such as osteogenesis imperfecta. An internal examination is generally not necessary, although sampling of tissue and/or blood for cytogenetic and DNA molecular diagnostic studies is required for specific diagnosis, and evaluation for osteogenesis imperfecta requires fetal tissue containing fibroblasts.[25] Plain radiographs may also identify abnormalities of ribs and/or vertebrae that were not visualized on ultrasound or routine external and internal pathologic examination and that may

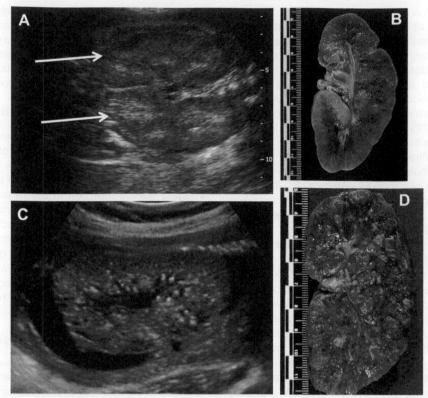

Fig. 2. Ultrasound does not always allow definitive diagnosis of fetal renal cystic disease, even although it is preferable to MR imaging for delineating renal anomalies. (*A*) Ultrasound, 28 weeks, showing enlarged bilateral echogenic kidneys (*arrows*), suggestive of autosomal recessive polycystic kidney disease (ARPKD). (*B*) Corresponding kidney from autopsy at 33 to 34 weeks, showing characteristic parenchymal features of confirmed ARPKD, confirmed by histology and molecular diagnosis. (*C*) Ultrasound, 22 weeks: bilaterally enlarged echogenic kidneys with no definite large cysts, diagnosed as probable ARPKD by 2 experienced radiologists. (*D*) Corresponding kidney from autopsy, showing histologically confirmed bilateral diffuse renal cystic dysplasia.

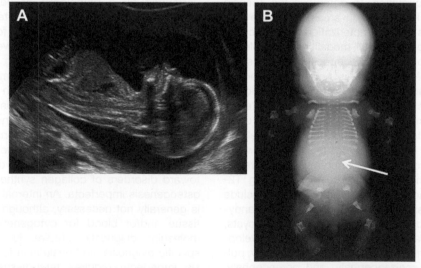

Fig. 3. Usefulness of plain radiographs to identify diagnostic features not visualized on antemortem ultrasound. Ultrasound (*A*) and postmortem plain radiograph (*B*) of a skeletal dysplasia diagnosed on plain radiography as achondrogenesis type 1b, later confirmed by molecular diagnostic studies. Note the absence of vertebral bodies (*arrow*) on the plain radiograph. (*Data from* Gilbert-Barnes E. Osteochondrodysplasias–Constitutional diseases of bone. In: Gilbert-Barnes E, editor. Potter's pathology of the fetus, infant and child, vol. 2. 2nd edition. Philadelphia: Mosby-Elsevier; 2007.)

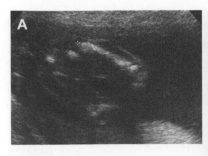
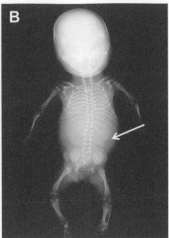
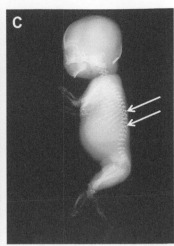

Fig. 4. Usefulness of plain radiographs to identify diagnostic features not visualized on antemortem ultrasound. Ultrasound (*A*) of humerus showing normal mineralization of the bones with no bowing. Postmortem plain radiograph frontal view (*B*) and lateral view (*C*) identified this as chondrodysplasia punctata because of the platyspondyly (*double arrows*) and the irregularity seen at the epiphyses in all long bones (*arrow*). This radiographic feature guided subsequent chemical and molecular diagnostic studies to diagnose X-linked chondrodysplasia punctata, also called Conradi-Hunermann type (CDPx2). (*Data from* Gilbert-Barnes E. Osteochondrodysplasias–Constitutional diseases of bone. In: Gilbert-Barnes E, editor. Potter's pathology of the fetus, infant & child, vol. 2. 2nd edition. Philadelphia: Mosby-Elsevier; 2007.)

allow more specific classification of a malformation complex, such as VACTERL association or sacral dysgenesis in diabetic fetopathy (**Fig. 5**). These radiographs are most easily obtained using freestanding specimen radiologic units designed for pathology laboratories.[13,26] Ready availability of specimen radiography equipment in the pathology laboratory allows routine plain-film radiography of all fetuses and infants before examination, because these studies do not interfere with diagnostic radiologic procedures or incur additional cost for radiology personnel and equipment. When clinical radiology facilities are used, test performance may be limited to those fetuses in which skeletal dysplasia is a clinical concern, or in which abnormalities are identified pathologically in which radiologic imaging would contribute diagnostically. At University of Washington Medical Center, fetal autopsy routinely includes postmortem radiography via Faxitron (Lincolnshire, IL, USA),[26] with standard anterior and lateral radiographs of the whole body, and detailed radiographs of specific areas of interest (eg, hands and feet) obtained if needed.

Postmortem computed tomography (CT) imaging can be used to evaluate skeletal abnormalities in the fetus or infant. CT imaging has been in wide use in the clinical setting for a longer time than MR imaging, and is less expensive and faster to perform. However, postmortem visualization of soft-tissue structures is poor,

precluding the use of postmortem CT scanning to replace internal autopsy examination. Thayyil and colleagues[3] have suggested that CT imaging with three-dimensional reconstruction could allow excellent visualization of bony structures, and substitute for plain-film radiography, although this has not been systematically evaluated. Plain-film radiography is less expensive and more accessible for most pathology laboratories.

Postmortem MR Imaging

Postmortem MR imaging has been used for nearly 2 decades, and its use and evaluation have expanded. Early studies focused on forensic evaluations in trauma. In fetal and infant autopsy, a primary focus has been the evaluation of structural abnormalities of the brain and CNS, because of the limitations of autopsy in this setting.

MR imaging is based on the presence of hydrogen nuclei (protons) in the water content of body tissues. In contrast to CT imaging, MR imaging provides excellent visualization of soft tissues, and poor delineation of bony structures. In the brain, differences in hydrogen ion content of the gray and white matter allows for particularly good delineation of internal structures.[7]

Pathologic examination of the fetal and infant brain poses unique challenges in part because of the high water content of the brain tissue, which limits the structural integrity, complicates removal

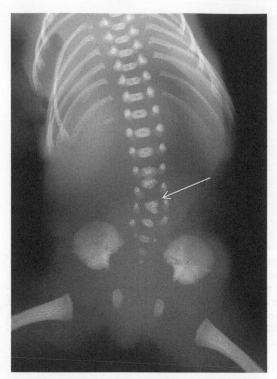

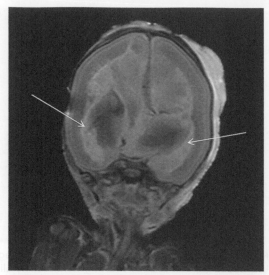

Fig. 6. Postmortem MR imaging, 21 weeks' gestation, showing massive ventriculomegaly (*arrows*), clearly differentiated from holoprosencephaly, which was the differential diagnosis by prenatal ultrasound.

Fig. 5. Usefulness of plain radiographs to identify diagnostic features not visualized on antemortem ultrasound. Identification of vertebral abnormalities (hemivertebrae [*arrow*]) as seen in VACTERL association and diabetic fetopathy. These abnormalities were not visualized on antemortem ultrasound. (*Data from* Siebert JR, Kapur Raj. Back and Perineum. In: Gilbert-Barnes E, editor. Potter's pathology of the fetus, infant and child, vol. 2. 2nd edition. Philadelphia: Mosby-Elsevier; 2007.)

and examination of the unfixed brain, and results in significant liquefaction after short periods of intrauterine demise. A major advantage of MR imaging is that it allows evaluation of the brain in situ, so as to minimize the damage and distortion that result from removal of the brain.

Examination in situ by MR imaging allows detailed delineation of the external and internal anatomy of the brain and spinal cord, allowing both the detection of developmental and acquired abnormalities and confirmation of normal anatomy. In addition to the ability to assess anatomic structures in situ, MR imaging is superior in the evaluation of ventricular size and configuration and assessing abnormalities of the posterior fossa, such as cysts, Dandy-Walker malformation complex, and cerebellar malformations (see **Fig. 1**; **Figs. 6** and **7**). Similarly, MR imaging provides excellent delineation of the structural anatomy of soft tissues of the limbs and of the internal organs of the chest and abdomen. The delineation of

abnormal fluid collections in body cavities and soft tissues (scalp, limbs) is excellent, allowing visualization of effusions, collections of blood and air in body cavities (hemo- and pneumothorax), soft-tissue edema, and masses. Many structural malformations can be clearly visualized, such as diaphragmatic hernia, teratomas, renal agenesis, situs inversus, bladder-outlet obstruction, and cystic renal disease. However, some structural abnormalities cannot be reliably identified, such as tracheoesophageal fistula, abnormalities of bowel rotation, and structural anomalies of the heart, particularly atrial and ventricular septal defects, and abnormalities of valves and outflow tracts and proximal great vessels.[27] Even when abnormalities of the bowel can be described in terms of the structural changes, the specific cause may not be delineated, as when dilated bowel suggests a distal obstruction. Processes that do not result in structural abnormalities, such as metabolic or infectious disease, may not be identified at MR imaging. Tissue changes related to postmortem autolysis (maceration) or decomposition may confound the interpretation of MR imaging, and infections and metabolic disease may not be identified.[2]

In early studies, postmortem MR imaging of the CNS was considered to have high sensitivity and specificity. For example, Griffiths and colleagues[28] reported a series of T2-weighted images in 40 fetuses and stillborn neonates, ranging from 14 to 42 weeks' gestational age, in which the brain and spinal cord were examined without formalin

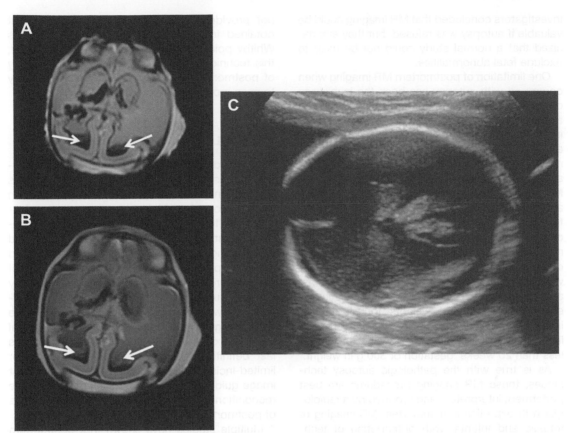

Fig. 7. Postmortem MR imaging: axial fluid-attenuated inversion recovery (*A*) and T2-weighted images (*B*), 24 weeks' gestation, showing massive bilateral intraventricular hemorrhage (*arrows*) in a fetus diagnosed with trisomy 21. Ultrasound (*C*) showed bilateral ventriculomegaly, but did not show any definite signs of hemorrhage.

fixation. In 8 cases, no structural information was obtained by pathologic examination of the unfixed brain. In 97% of the 32 pathologically examined cases, there was agreement with the MR imaging, giving a sensitivity of 100% and a specificity of 92% for MR imaging. However, other studies have been more measured in their evaluation. Cohen and colleagues[7] described the results of postmortem MR imaging (1.5-T fast spin echo with T2-weighted images) of the CNS in 90 perinatal autopsies, ranging from 13 to 41 weeks' gestation, including both terminations of pregnancy and intrauterine fetal demises. In 79% of the cases, the quality of the MR images was equivalent to or better than the autopsy, and in 21%, the MR imaging quality was inferior to that of autopsy. In 60% of the cases, there was complete agreement between the MR imaging and autopsy of the CNS. However, in 13% of cases, autopsy CNS morphology was clearly superior. If the information obtained from the complete autopsy was compared with the MR imaging, autopsy allowed

identification of the cause of death or ascertainment of malformation in 37% of cases, and in 27% of cases, MR imaging added valuable information to the autopsy findings. However, if MR imaging had been the only information available and autopsy had not been performed, the investigators asserted that valuable information would have been lost in 71% of cases. However, in this study, MR imaging was limited to the CNS only, so that the comparison of the MR imaging results with those of the complete autopsy is misleading. A similar study by Alderliestan and colleagues[4] assessed 26 cases in which whole-body MR imaging was performed using clinical MR imaging and T1- and T2-weighted sequences. Only 56% of malformations identified by complete autopsy were detected by MR imaging, and sensitivity was best for CNS abnormalities. The low diagnostic accuracy was attributed to the small number of CNS abnormalities in their group and the evaluation of MR imaging in isolation from other evaluations, including external examination. The investigators concluded that MR imaging could be valuable if autopsy was refused, but they emphasized that a normal study could not be used to exclude fetal abnormalities.

One limitation of postmortem MR imaging when compared with autopsy has been the inability to determine the weights of organs, important in assessment of pathologic processes such as intrauterine growth restriction or specific organ abnormalities. To address this deficiency, techniques have been developed that allow relatively accurate estimation of organ weight based on MR imaging volumetric determinations. Thayyil and colleagues[29] used a semiautomated method for organ weight estimation using three-dimensional volume reconstructions after post-mortem whole-body MR imaging using a 1.5-T clinical scanner and three-dimensional T2-weighted sequence. In 65 fetuses, newborns, and children, there was excellent correlation of estimated and actual weights for all organs, including brain, liver, spleen, lungs, heart, and liver, although accuracy was lower with fetuses less than 20 weeks' gestation or 300 g in weight.

As is true with the pathologic autopsy techniques, these MR imaging procedures are best performed, interpreted, and reported by a radiologist with expertise in antemortem MR imaging of fetuses and infants, with optimization of techniques as required by fetal size, preservation, and anomalies. Most studies have used standard 1.5-T MR imaging with T2-weighted images, as in clinical MR imaging, and have optimized techniques by using small coils or other modifications to increase image quality. However, these techniques have been satisfactory only for larger fetuses weighing more than 300 g (approximately 24 weeks' gestation). Thayyil and colleagues[30] used high-field MR imaging at 9.4 T, with T2-weighted scans, and showed that this technique could be used in smaller fetuses, showing good tissue contrast, spatial resolution, and image quality, with a scan time of less than 2 hours. In a study of 18 fetuses with median gestational age of 16 weeks (range 11–22 weeks) and median weight of 59 g (range 5–400 g), high-field MR imaging identified all abnormalities detected at autopsy, even although 76% of the fetuses were either macerated or mummified. With intrauterine retention of less than 1 week, diagnostic images were obtained in all cases, and with intrauterine retention of more than 1 week, diagnostic images of the brain were obtained in 50% and of other organs in 25%. In contrast, diagnostic images were obtained in only 14% using conventional MR imaging at 1.5 T, and diagnostic information was obtained by autopsy in 24%. Autopsy did

not provide additional information beyond that obtained from 9.4-T imagining in any case. As Whitby points out in the accompanying editorial, this technique is a major advance in the quality of postmortem imaging, and may pave the way to even more detailed evaluation.[31]

MINIMAL POSTMORTEM EXAMINATION (MINIMALLY INVASIVE AUTOPSY)

Thayyil and colleagues[10] defined a minimally invasive autopsy as "an autopsy process that includes information from all noninvasive postmortem investigations (which) include external examination of the fetus, placental histopathology, cytogenetic investigations, postmortem radiography, and MR imaging, and exclude invasive dissection, and macroscopic or microscopic examination of visceral organs." Other definitions of minimally invasive autopsy include all noninvasive evaluations, as well as invasive investigations of more limited degree than that used in the conventional autopsy examination of the trunk and brain. This last definition includes percutaneous-needle or limited-incision biopsies, both with and without image guidance. These last definitions reflect the recognition of the advantages and disadvantages of postmortem MR imaging.

Multiple studies have shown that postmortem MR imaging can provide internal structural anatomic delineation that is often equivalent to that of internal pathologic examination. In some cases, MR imaging can provide information superior to that of traditional autopsy, particularly for intracranial and cerebral abnormalities, and in the setting of postmortem maceration. Images can be retained as a permanent record, although autopsy materials such as photographs, histologic slides, and retained tissue (either processed, frozen, or fixed) can also be retained for further investigation. Disadvantages of postmortem MR imaging include the availability of instrumentation, cost, and the requirement for skilled technicians and interpretation by a radiologist with expertise in both fetal and infant disease and postmortem changes. However, the major disadvantage of MR imaging is that specific etiologic diagnosis often requires histopathologic examination, particularly important in the assessment of infection, ischemia, hypoxia, and metabolic disorders, which may present structural changes similar to those seen with purely developmental or anatomic anomalies.[6,8,9]

One approach to the need for histologic evaluation has been to use limited histologic evaluation of organs other than the brain in concert with postmortem MR imaging of the brain to formulate a most probable diagnosis. Nicholl and colleagues[32] reported a small series of 6 neonatal deaths in which encephalopathy was a prominent feature. MR imaging was used in concert with biopsies of tissues other than the brain and other data to formulate a diagnosis, based on the integration of all information, and similar to diagnostic evaluation in living patients. This type of evaluation has the same limitations of any set of antemortem diagnoses, in that the absence of histologic evaluation of the diseased organ precludes the most definitive diagnosis.

Others have proposed use of image-guided percutaneous biopsies, following high-quality MR imaging, to avoid open dissection of the body. However, studies using biopsy without image guidance have been disappointing. Breeze and colleagues[33] assessed the feasibility of using percutaneous-needle biopsy to obtain tissue, and had a success rate for obtaining tissue of less than 50%, not related to time to biopsy after death, gestational age, body weight, or user experience. Tissue samples were most often successful in lung and liver, and less frequently in heart, kidney, adrenal, thymus, and spleen, with histologically adequate tissue obtained in fewer than half of fetal renal biopsies. There was poor diagnostic accuracy when compared with histologic diagnoses at autopsy, and the investigators described that no histologic diagnoses determined by autopsy were identified by needle biopsy. In a follow-up study,[5] the comparability and clinical value of a combination of postmortem MR imaging and percutaneous fetal organ biopsies (so-called minimally invasive autopsy) was compared with conventional or traditional fetal autopsy, in 44 fetal fetuses with a mean age of 24 weeks. A pediatric radiologist and neuroradiologist reported the imaging, percutaneous organ biopsy was performed by a clinician with a Tenino cutting biopsy needle using external landmarks but no imaging guidance, and autopsy was performed by a pediatric histopathologist. Review of the biopsy histology was performed by a different pediatric histopathologist, and all the participants were blinded to the results of the other specialty's studies. The results of all ancillary studies (such as karyotype, microbiological cultures or evaluations, infectious serology, plain radiography, and placental pathology) were considered to be common to both the conventional and the minimally invasive evaluation, and the modalities were compared in terms of discordant information and diagnostic usefulness. In 21 cases, the conventional and minimally invasive autopsies provided equivalent diagnostic information, and in 21 cases, the conventional autopsy provided superior diagnostic information. In 2 cases, the minimally invasive autopsy provided superior diagnostic information, and both were cases in which postmortem autolysis precluded brain evaluation. In 73% (32 cases), the minimally invasive autopsy provided information of at least equivalent clinical significance to the conventional autopsy. In no case did the addition of percutaneous biopsy without imaging guidance identify information of additional clinical significance. In this setting, the investigators concluded that the value of percutaneous biopsy was not proved.

One novel approach to postmortem diagnosis was proposed by Fan and colleagues,[34] in which surgeon-performed thoracoscopy and laparoscopy was used in the postmortem setting, along with endoscopic examination of great vessels. Limited incision and biopsy was performed in 4 of 18 cases. No radiologic imaging was used in this study, in which diagnostic accuracy was said to be 94%, when compared with conventional autopsy. However, this type of minimally invasive tissue procurement procedure might be used in conjunction with radiologic imaging to obtain tissue samples for histologic evaluation and more definitive diagnosis.

In the most recent review of this subject, Thayyil and colleagues[10] systematically reviewed all published studies on the accuracy of postmortem MR imaging in fetuses, children, and adults, and identified only 9 studies from which data could be extracted. The diagnostic accuracy of postmortem MR imaging in fetuses for determining the cause of death or most clinically significant abnormality had a sensitivity of 69% (with a 95% confidence interval of 56%–80%) and a specificity of 95% (with a 95% confidence interval of 23%–94%). Accuracy was poorer in children and adults. However, the investigators described the published studies as small and poorly designed, and to be inadequate to evaluate the diagnostic accuracy, or other factors such as acceptability by families and economic feasibility of postmortem MR imaging.

INVESTIGATION OF FETAL AND PERINATAL DEATHS: AN INTEGRATED APPROACH

There is general agreement that postmortem MR imaging is a valuable component of a death investigation, and although unlikely to completely replace the traditional autopsy, it can be used as part of a minimally invasive autopsy in an integrated approach to postmortem diagnosis in fetal and perinatal deaths.[3,31] Although traditional autopsy with histopathologic evaluation of tissues is still considered to be the gold standard for death investigation, the best approach uses a multidisciplinary team to work with a family to provide diagnostic information, respecting a family's desires about the handling of the deceased fetus or infant's body. Appropriate noninvasive procedures could be used in every fetal death, with postmortem imaging, tissue sampling, and traditional autopsy recommended and used based on interdisciplinary consultation with providers from maternal-fetal medicine, genetics and genetic counseling, pathology and laboratory medicine, and others specialties as required by the specific case (eg, pediatric cardiology and nephrology).[31] This system for postmortem diagnosis recapitulates medical diagnosis in the setting of complex diseases, in which multiple specialists interact to formulate diagnostic and therapeutic plans for patients. Similar programs are seen in multidisciplinary tumor boards for malignancies, which integrate specialists from oncology, surgery, pathology, and radiology, with support for the patient by representatives from social work, psychology, and spiritual care. In the setting of fetal/perinatal death investigation, the specialist evaluation group would interact not only in the setting of prenatal diagnosis and planning for the death investigation but also in the diagnostic evaluation and integration of data from all modalities.

SUMMARY

Although traditional pathologic autopsy is still considered the gold standard for investigation of fetal death, radiographic imaging can be an important adjunct to any fetal and perinatal autopsy in all cases. Much important information in a fetal/perinatal death investigation is provided by ancillary studies, which include external examination of the body by a pathologist with expertise in fetal and infant pathology; detailed placental examination; plain-film radiography; cytogenetics and molecular diagnostic evaluation; and fetal and maternal microbiological and serologic studies. Antenatal ultrasound, and in some cases MR imaging, can assist in directing and modifying the autopsy examination. The use of postmortem MR imaging, in combination with ancillary studies, can provide information of equivalent clinical significance in some, but not all, deaths. The major limitation of a noninvasive, imaging-only postmortem investigation is the absence of macroscopic visualization of organs and histologic evaluation of organs and tissues. Development of minimally invasive tissue-procurement procedures that can be used in conjunction with noninvasive MR imaging should be encouraged, as should the optimization of postmortem MR imaging

techniques for small fetuses and for the differentiation of postmortem from antemortem processes. Minimally invasive or noninvasive autopsy does not provide sufficient data to accurately determine cause of death or major pathologic abnormalities in all cases. Large-scale, well-designed studies assessing the value of and appropriate methodologies for minimally invasive autopsy may help to determine how best to use these postmortem procedures in a given death. Optimal use requires integrated systems for planning and interpretation of diagnostic modalities, using providers from multiple specialties, to provide optimal diagnosis, management, and counseling in the setting of fetal and perinatal disease.

ACKNOWLEDGMENTS

Special thanks to Jessica Norberg and Layne Harrington, in University of Washington Medical Center (UWMC) Autopsy and After Death Services, for excellent photographic assistance; Virginia Lore and Aurora Bender, UWMC Anatomic Pathology, for assistance with the manuscript; and Marie Leonard, UWMC Radiology, for assistance with the figures.

REFERENCES

1. Gordijn SJ, Erwich JJ, Khong TY. The perinatal autopsy: pertinent issues in multicultural Western Europe. Eur J Obstet Gynecol Reprod Biol 2007; 132(1):3–7.
2. Jones R. Post-mortem imaging–an update. In: Kirkham N, Shepherd NA, editors. Progress in pathology, vol. 7. Cambridge (UK): Cambridge University Press; 2007. p. 199–220.
3. Thayyil S, Chitty LS, Robertson NJ, et al. Minimally invasive fetal postmortem examination using magnetic resonance imaging and computerised tomography: current evidence and practical issues. Prenat Diagn 2010;30(8):713–8.
4. Alderliesten ME, Peringa J, van der Hulst VP, et al. Perinatal mortality: clinical value of postmortem magnetic resonance imaging compared with autopsy in routine obstetric practice. BJOG 2003; 110(4):378–82.
5. Breeze AC, Jessop FA, Set PA, et al. The clinical value and comparability of a minimally-invasive fetal autopsy using magnetic resonance imaging and percutaneous organ biopsies in comparison to conventional autopsy. Ultrasound Obstet Gynecol 2011;37(3):317–23.
6. Brookes JS, Hagmann C. MRI in fetal necropsy. J Magn Reson Imaging 2006;24(6):1221–8.
7. Cohen MC, Paley MN, Griffiths PD, et al. Less invasive autopsy: benefits and limitations of the use of

magnetic resonance imaging in the perinatal post-mortem. Pediatr Dev Pathol 2008;11(1):1–9.

8. Huisman T. Magnetic resonance imaging: an alternative to autopsy in neonatal death? Semin Neonatol 2004;9(4):347–53.

9. Whitby EH, Paley MN, Cohen M, et al. Postmortem MR imaging of the fetus: an adjunct or a replacement for conventional autopsy? Semin Fetal Neonatal Med 2005;10(5):475–83.

10. Thayyil S, Chandrasekaran M, Chitty LS, et al. Diagnostic accuracy of post-mortem magnetic resonance imaging in fetuses, children and adults: a systematic review. Eur J Radiol 2010;75(1):e142–e148.

11. Washington State Department of Health. Washington state death and fetal death registration handbook. Olympia (WA): Center for Health Statistics; 2004.

12. Siebert JR. Perinatal, fetal, and embryonic autopsy. In: Gilbert-Barness E, editor. 2nd edition, Potter's pathology of the fetus, infant, and child, vol. 1. Mosby-Elsevier; 2007. p. 695–740. Chapter 16.

13. Finkbeiner WE, Ursell PC, Davis RL. Autopsy pathology: a manual and atlas. 2nd edition. Philadelphia: Saunders-Elsevier; 2009. p. 81–91.

14. Gilbert-Barness E, Debich-Spicer DE. Handbook of pediatric autopsy pathology. Totowa (NJ): Humana Press; 2005.

15. Kapur RP. Use of ancillary tests in perinatal pathology. In: Gilbert-Barness E, editor. Potter's pathology of the fetus, infant, and child, vol. 1. Mosby-Elsevier; 2007. p. 871–84. Chapter 19.

16. Kapur RP. Practicing pediatric pathology without a microscope. Mod Pathol 2001;14(3):229–35.

17. Tellefsen C, Vogt C. How important is placental examination in cases of perinatal deaths? Pediatr Dev Pathol 2010. [Epub ahead of print].

18. Online Mendelian Inheritance in Man. Available at: http://www.ncbi.nlm.nih.gov/omim. Accessed February 25, 2011.

19. GeneClinics. Available at: http://www.ncbi.nlm.nih.gov/sites/GeneTests/?db=GeneTests. Accessed February 25, 2011.

20. Akgun H, Basbug M, Ozgun M, et al. Correlation between prenatal ultrasound and fetal autopsy findings in fetal anomalies terminated in the second trimester. Prenat Diagn 2007;27(5):457–62.

21. Phillips JJ, Mahony BS, Siebert JR, et al. Dandy-Walker malformation complex: correlation between ultrasonographic diagnosis and postmortem neuropathology. Obstet Gynecol 2006;107(3):685–93.

22. Gupta P, Kumar S, Sharma R, et al. The role of magnetic resonance imaging in fetal renal anomalies. Int J Gynaecol Obstet 2010;111(3):209–12.

23. Dean A, Whitby E. Contribution of antenatal magnetic resonance imaging to diagnostic neuropathology. Curr Diagn Pathol 2007;13(3):171–9.

24. Dighe M, Fligner C, Cheng E, et al. Fetal skeletal dysplasia: an approach to diagnosis with illustrative cases. Radiographics 2008;28(4):1061–77.

25. Collagen Diagnostic Laboratory. 2010. Available at: http://www.pathology.washington.edu/clinical/collagen/. Accessed February 25, 2011.

26. Available at: http://www.faxitron.com/medical/pathology.html. Accessed February 25, 2011.

27. Breeze AC, Cross JJ, Hackett GA, et al. Use of a confidence scale in reporting postmortem fetal magnetic resonance imaging. Ultrasound Obstet Gynecol 2006;28(7):918–24.

28. Griffiths PD, Variend D, Evans M, et al. Postmortem MR imaging of the fetal and stillborn central nervous system. AJNR Am J Neuroradiol 2003;24(1):22–7.

29. Thayyil S, Schievano S, Robertson N, et al. A semi-automated method for non-invasive internal organ weight estimation by post-mortem magnetic resonance imaging in fetuses, newborns and children. Eur J Radiol 2009;72(2):321–6.

30. Thayyil S, Cleary JO, Sebire NJ, et al. Post-mortem examination of human fetuses: a comparison of whole-body high-field MRI at 9.4 T with conventional MRI and invasive autopsy. Lancet 2009;374:467–75.

31. Whitby E. Minimally invasive autopsy. Lancet 2009;374(9688):432–3.

32. Nicholl RM, Balasubramaniam VP, Urquhart DS, et al. Postmortem brain MRI with selective tissue biopsy as an adjunct to autopsy following neonatal encephalopathy. Eur J Paediatr Neurol 2007;11(3):167–74.

33. Breeze AC, Jessop FA, Whitehead AL, et al. Feasibility of percutaneous organ biopsy as part of a minimally invasive perinatal autopsy. Virchows Arch 2008;452(2):201–7.

34. Fan J, Tong D, Poon J, et al. Multimodality minimally invasive autopsy–a feasible and accurate approach to post-mortem examination. Forensic Sci Int 2010;195(1–3):93–8.

Imaging of Twin Pregnancies

Mariam Moshiri, MD

KEYWORDS

• Twins • Prenatal • Ultrasonography

DETERMINATION OF CHORIONICITY

Twin pregnancies account for approximately 10 in 1000 live births in the United States (variable based on geographic location). The incidence of twinning has been increasing in developing countries because of 2 factors: use of fertility treatment and advanced maternal age. The rate of twinning is 3.8 times higher with assisted reproduction than in the general population. Multiple gestations account for 10% of all perinatal morbidity and mortality. Complications in twin gestation are similar to those of singleton gestations but occur with higher frequency. In addition, twinning is associated with unique fetal complications and higher frequency of maternal complications.[1–3] In general population, increasing maternal age, parity, and positive family history are factors that can increase the rate of twinning. The paternal history has no effect on the twinning rates. The maternal race is also a factor, and the incidence of twin gestation increases incrementally if the mother is of Asian, Caucasian, and African American background.[4]

Approximately 70% of twin pregnancies are dizygotic and are the result of the fertilization of 2 separate ova, which form 2 separate zygotes. Because these twins have different genetic material they can be of different sex. Dizygotic twins are also referred to as fraternal twins. Dizygotic twinning can also originate from a single fertilized ovum. When the zygote divides before the fourth day of fertilization (before chorion differentiation), the pregnancy would be dichorionic and diamniotic. This condition occurs in about 25% of monozygotic twinning.[5] Each zygote develops independently and forms its own blastocyst, which implants in the uterus approximately 7 days after fertilization. Each blastocyst gives rise to the placenta, chorionic membrane, amnion, yolk sac, umbilical cord, and fetus. Therefore, all dizygotic twins are dichorionic (2 placentas) and diamniotic.[6] Incidence of monozygotic twins is less common, accounting for 30% of twin pregnancies. The incidence of monozygotic twinning is independent of any maternal factors, such as race, age, or parity. However, recent studies report that the rate of monozygotic twinning following assisted reproductive techniques is between 2 and 12 times higher than that of the general population.[2] Because monozygotic twins are formed from the same cell line, they share the same genetic material and are of the same sex. They are also referred to as identical twins. Monozygotic twinning is the result of very early split of a single zygote. When the zygote divides between days 4 and 8 of fertilization (before amnion differentiation), the pregnancy would be monochorionic diamniotic. This condition occurs in about 75% of monozygotic twins. Division of a zygote 8 days after fertilization (after amnion formation) results in monochorionic monoamniotic pregnancy. Cleavage of the embryonic disk more than 13 days after fertilization is usually incomplete and results in conjoined twins. All conjoined twins are monozygotic monoamniotic (Fig. 1).[4,6]

Twin pregnancy–related complications have variable presentation and severity depending on the type of twinning, and therefore, they are of outmost importance to clinicians in the management of such pregnancies. Sonographic assessment of chorionicity and amnionicity of multiple

The author has nothing to disclose.
Department of Radiology, University of Washington School of Medicine, University of Washington Medical Center, 1959 NE Pacific Street, Box 357115, Seattle, WA 98195, USA
E-mail address: moshiri@u.washington.edu

Ultrasound Clin 6 (2011) 119–132
doi:10.1016/j.cult.2011.01.006

ultrasound.theclinics.com

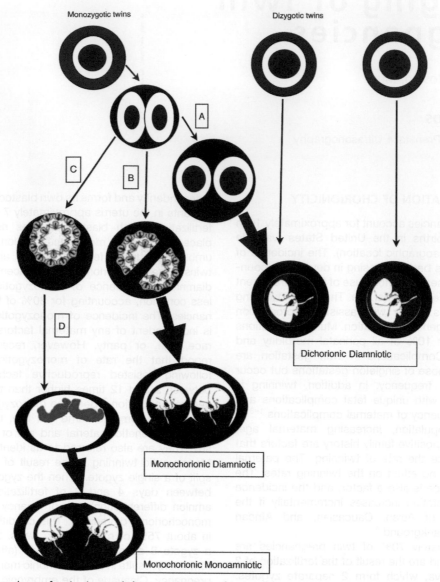

Fig. 1. Embryology of twinning and the various types of twins.

gestations is most accurate in the first trimester of pregnancy.[7]

Sonographic assessment of the number of gestational sacs is an accurate method for predicting chorionicity between the 6th and 10th weeks of gestation. Determination of chorionicity before the sixth week of gestation can result in 15% inaccuracy.[8] During the 6th to 10th gestational weeks, the fluid-filled gestational sac identified on ultrasonography is predominantly the chorionic cavity. However, as the first trimester progresses, the amniotic cavity enlarges, fills, and obliterates the chorionic cavity. Therefore, in the early weeks of first trimester, the number of

gestational sacs equals the chorionicity number (**Fig. 2**). Between the 10th and 14th weeks of gestation, visualization of the twin peak sign (also called the lambda sign) is a reliable predictor of dichorionic pregnancy (**Figs. 3** and **4**). This sign represents the extension of placental villi into the potential space that is formed between the opposing 2-layer combination of amnion and chorion from each gestational sac. In a monochorionic pregnancy, only a single layer of continuous chorion exists, which hinders growth of the villi between the 2 opposing layers of amnion (**Figs. 5** and **6**). This hindrance results in the appearance of only a thin membrane separating the 2 fetuses.[9]

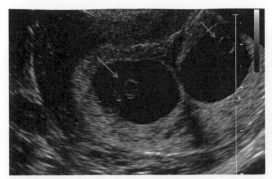

Fig. 2. Early dichorionic diamniotic twin pregnancy. Note that 2 sacs are compatible with dichorionic pregnancy and 2 separate yolk sacs (*arrows*) are compatible with diamniotic pregnancy.

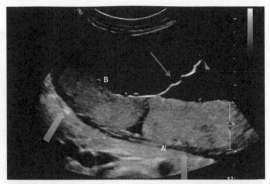

Fig. 4. Third trimester dichorionic diamniotic twin pregnancy. Note 2 separate placental masses (*large arrows*); however, the membrane between the 2 gestational sacs appears thinner (*small arrow*) as it gets stretched with advancing gestational age. A and B each refer to a separate placenta.

DETERMINATION OF AMNIONICITY

Because the amnion forms after the chorion, dichorionicity implies diamnionicity. Visualization of 2 embryos in 1 gestational sac challenges amnionicity determination because the pregnancy is monochorionic but could be monoamniotic or diamniotic. Identification of the yolk sacs can be helpful in this regard. Monochorionic diamniotic gestations are always associated with 2 yolk sacs. Monochorionic monoamniotic gestations are associated with either 1 yolk sac or, more rarely, a divided one (**Fig. 7**). Therefore, visualization of a single yolk sac in a twin gestation before 8 weeks of pregnancy should prompt a follow-up examination for re-evaluation of the number of yolk sacs or the number of amnions.[10] Between 10th and 14th weeks of gestation, the appearance of a single thin membrane without the twin peak sign is a reliable indicator of diamniotic gestation. This sign is sometimes referred to as the "T"

sign.[11] In summary, the number of yolk sacs equals the amnionicity number.

OTHER HELPFUL OBSERVATIONS

If the fetuses are of different sex, then the pregnancy is dizygotic, dichorionic, and diamniotic. If 2 separate placental masses are seen, then the pregnancy is dichorionic and diamniotic. This observation, however, becomes less reliable in the later gestation period because the 2 separate placental masses could fuse because of their size (**Table 1**).

PITFALLS

As the pregnancy progresses, all membranes become thinner, and therefore, the twin peak

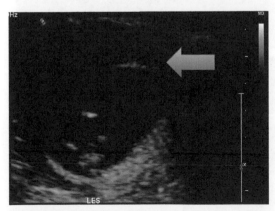

Fig. 3. First trimester dichorionic diamniotic twin pregnancy. Note the thick membrane between the 2 sacs (twin peak sign) (*arrow*), suggesting a dichorionic diamniotic twin pregnancy.

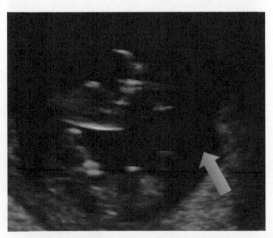

Fig. 5. Early monochorionic diamniotic twin pregnancy. Note the thin membrane between the 2 fetuses (*arrow*), suggesting a diamniotic pregnancy.

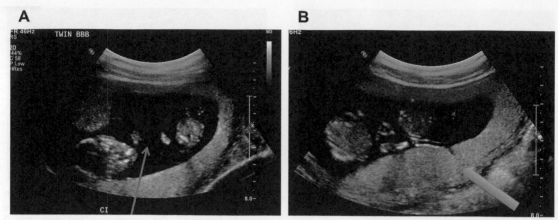

Fig. 6. Monochorionic diamniotic twin pregnancy in later gestation. (*A*) A thin membrane between the twins (*arrow*) suggesting a diamniotic pregnancy. (*B*) A single placental mass is seen between the twins (*arrow*) suggesting a monochorionic pregnancy.

sign may not be reliably observed in the later gestational age. Also later in the gestation, the fetal gender maybe difficult to assess. It may also be difficult to determine whether the placental mass is composed of 2 adjacent fused placentas or the pregnancy is actually supported by a single placenta.

COMPLICATIONS

Twin gestations exhibit 3 to 7 times higher rates of perinatal morbidity and mortality than singleton gestations. This increase is mostly due to increased rates of fetal growth restriction, as well as structural and chromosomal fetal anomalies, some of which are unique to twin gestations.[12]

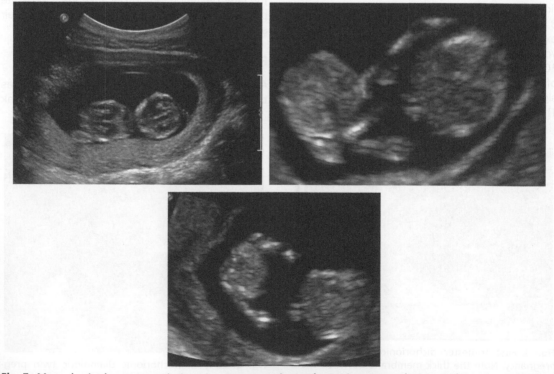

Fig. 7. Monochorionic monoamniotic twin pregnancy. A membrane is not seen between the twins, with close approximation of the fetal limbs, suggesting a monochorionic monoamniotic twin pregnancy.

Table 1
Ultrasonographic findings in various types of twins

Twin Type	Number of Chorions	Number of Yolk Sacs	Intervening Membranes	Fetal Gender	Placenta
Dichorionic Diamniotic	2	2	Thick, twin peak sign	Could be different or same	2 separate masses, could fuse later
Monochorionic Diamniotic	1	2	Thin	Same	1
Monochorionic Monoamniotic	1	1	None	Same	1

The rate and prevalence of complications increase from a dichorionic diamniotic (di-di) to a monochorionic diamniotic (mono-di) to a monochorionic monoamniotic (mono-mono) pregnancy.

Fetal Structural Anomalies

Structural anomalies occur more frequently in twins, affecting approximately 6% of diamniotic and 20% of monoamniotic pregnancies.[13] They usually affect 1 twin but account for most neonatal deaths. Therefore, twin gestations should be carefully assessed by ultrasonography. If a severe anomaly is detected, selective fetal reduction by umbilical cord occlusion could be discussed with the parents.[13]

Placenta, Amniotic Fluid Index, and Umbilical Cord

In dichorionic diamniotic twins, there are separate placentas supporting each twin. In some instances, the placentas could have an adjacent implantation site and could fuse later in gestation and appear as 1 placental mass. The remaining twin types have a single placenta supporting both twins. For all 3 categories of twinning, there is an increased risk of placenta previa and placental abruption.

Vasa previa also occurs with increased frequency in twin gestations.[14] The fetal vessels, which cross the internal cervical os, are at increased risk for tearing during labor resulting in fetal exsanguination. Velamentous cord insertion is seen with increased frequency in monochorionic pregnancies, which is associated with increased risk of discordant birth weights.[15]

In monoamniotic pregnancies, the umbilical cords typically insert close to one another, with multiple large-caliber anastomoses connecting the stem vessels of both twins. Therefore, cord entanglement and cord fusion are complications unique to monoamniotic twins. The entangled cords are believed to result in vascular compromise in 1 or both twins, which could lead to fetal demise.[15,16] Therefore, systematic evaluation of the umbilical cord by ultrasonography and color Doppler is imperative. Henrich and Tutschek[17] suggest the use of 2-dimensional and 3-dimensional (D) color Doppler imaging for accurate assessment. On color Doppler imaging, a branching pattern of cord vessels is noted in the region of the knot. On pulsed Doppler imaging, the end systolic notch in the umbilical artery is abnormal, which may reflect hemodynamic alterations in vessels narrowed by knotting. A recent study by Dias and colleagues[18] reviewed 32 monoamniotic twins and found that umbilical cord entanglement was present in all monoamniotic twins and that the actual cause of perinatal mortality was attributed to other complications. However, the small size of the study group warrants further investigation before any change in management.

Cord fusion is another umbilical cord anomaly unique to monoamniotic pregnancies. The fetal umbilical cords fuse a short distance from the placental insertion, resulting in a Y-shaped or forked appearance. Color Doppler ultrasonography can assist in distinguishing this entity from a cord entanglement.[18]

Amniotic fluid index is an unreliable measure of the amniotic fluid volume in multiple gestations, and the single deepest pocket method is used instead.[19] In this method, polyhydramnios is indicated when the deepest vertical pocket of fluid is greater than 8 cm and oligohydramnios when the deepest vertical pocket of fluid is less than 2 cm.[13] Asymmetric distribution of amniotic fluid volume in monochorionic twins could be a sign of complications, such as twin-twin transfusion syndrome (TTTS), twin reversed arterial perfusion sequence, or twin embolization syndrome.[20]

Twin-Twin Transfution Syndrome

TTTS is uniquely seen in 8% to 10% of monochorionic pregnancies.[21] It is usually diagnosed between 16 and 26 weeks of gestation and is the most important cause of perinatal mortality and morbidity in monochorionic twins. TTTS is believed to be caused by intertwin vascular anastomoses and imbalance of perfusion across the placenta. One twin is considered the donor, which partly transfuses the recipient twin. The donor twin demonstrates oliguria, hypovolemia, and oligohydramnios, whereas the recipient twin demonstrates polyuria, hypervolemia, and polyhydramnios.[13]

The sonographic diagnosis is based on the strict criteria of amniotic fluid discordance. TTTS occurs less frequently in monochorionic monoamniotic twins, and it is more difficult to diagnose because the asymmetry in amniotic fluid distribution is not apparent. The twin growth is also usually asymmetric, with more than 20% difference in estimated fetal weight. Severe discordance suggests significant unequal placental sharing or the presence of fetal anomalies in the smaller twin. Presence of echogenic bowel in the donor twin could suggest fetal hypoxia.[21,22]

Sonographic evaluation of TTTS is complex. Screening for TTTS should begin in the first trimester when amnionicity and chorionicity are determined. If there is an abnormal fetal nuchal translucency, then the fetal ductus venosus should be assessed. Abnormal flow in the ductus venosus along with a single placental mass and abnormal nuchal translucency may identify twins at risk for TTTS and warrants close follow-up ultrasonographic examinations.[23]

Ultrasonographic findings of TTTS include asymmetric distribution of amniotic fluid with oligohydramnios in 1 fetus (deepest pocket <2 cm) and polyhydramnios in the other fetus (deepest pocket >8 cm) (Fig. 8). The recipient twin can exhibit signs of fetal hydrops and high cardiac output. The twins can also exhibit a discordant growth of 20% or more as assessed by estimated fetal weights. Doppler ultrasonography can demonstrate arteriovenous anastomoses on the placental surface.[21,22]

Doppler ultrasonography is used to demonstrate hemodynamic changes in vascular flow related to TTTS (Fig. 9). These changes include absent or reversal of end diastolic flow in the umbilical artery of the donor twin; pulsatile flow in the umbilical vein, implying impending heart failure; reversal of flow in the ductus venosus, implying cardiac decompensation; and reversal of flow in the inferior vena cava.[23]

Quintero and colleagues[22] have described a staging system that is clinically used to grade the severity of TTTS and predict pregnancy outcome. The various stages are as follows:

Stage 1: donor bladder visible, normal Doppler findings
Stage 2: donor bladder empty, normal Doppler findings
Stage 3: donor bladder empty, abnormal Doppler findings
Stage 4: hydrops in recipient
Stage 5: demise of 1 or both twins.

Untreated TTTS is associated with extremely high morbidity and mortality rates. Recently, several studies have focused on identification of

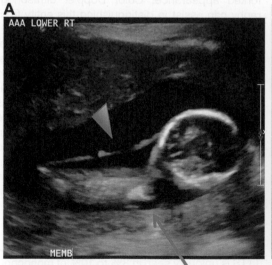
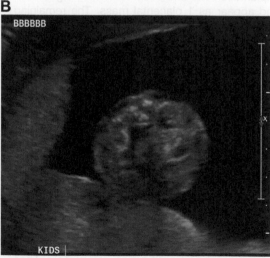

Fig. 8. TTTS. Ultrasonographic images showing monochorionic diamniotic twins (thin membrane, *arrowhead*). There is shunting of blood from twin A to twin B as seen by polyhydramnios in twin B (*B*) and oligohydramnios in twin A (*A*). Note the thin membrane (*arrow*) between the 2 twins.

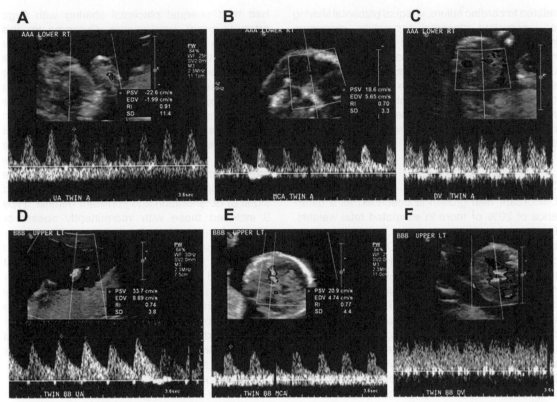

Fig. 9. Doppler imaging in TTTS. Monochorionic diamniotic twins. Normal flow is seen in twin B in the umbilical artery (UA) (*A*), middle cerebral artery (MCA) (*B*), and ductus venosus (DV) (*C*); however, there is decreased diastolic flow in UA (*D*), normal flow in MCA (*E*), and partial reversal of flow in DV (*F*) of twin A. EDV, end diastolic velocity; PSV, peak systolic velocity; RI, resistive index.

sonographic markers that could forecast the development of TTTS. Sebire and colleagues[24] found that pregnancies with increased nuchal translucency thickness in the first trimester and folding of the intertwin membrane in the second trimester are at increased risk of developing TTTS. Also presence of velamentous cord insertion and inability of ultrasonography to detect arteriovenous anastomosis have been commonly found in pregnancies with TTTS.[23]

Sueters and colleagues[23] reported that biweekly ultrasonographic examinations with special attention to the amniotic fluid compartments of both fetuses, combined with detailed patient instructions to report onset of symptoms resulted in timely diagnosis of all TTTS subjects in their study and appeared as a safe program to monitor those pregnancies at risk for TTTS. Lewi and colleagues[25] conducted a study to determine the value of ultrasonographic examination in the first trimester and at 16 weeks to predict fetal complications of monochorionic diamniotic pregnancies. They found that significant predictors in the first trimester were the difference in fetal crown-rump

length and discordant amniotic fluid. At 16 weeks, significant predictors were the difference in abdominal circumference, discordant amniotic fluid, and discordant cord insertion. The investigators determined that risk assessment in the first trimester and at 16 weeks detected 29% and 48% of cases with complicated fetal outcome with a false-positive rate of 3% and 6%, respectively. Combined first trimester and 16 week assessment identified 58% of fetal complications with a false-positive rate of 8%.[25] Monochorionic twins are at a higher risk for congenital anomalies, including heart disease, and discordant fetal growth.

Fetoscopic laser coagulation of the vascular anastomoses is the best mode of treatment currently available. Laser coagulation results in better survival rates and lesser rates of neurologic morbidity in the twins compared with serial amnioreductions.[26] Long-term developmental delays can occur in about 15% of surviving fetuses.[27]

Fetal loss is attributed to intrauterine fetal demise of 1 twin, most commonly occurring within the first postoperative week. This loss is likely related to cardiac failure, unequal placental sharing or incomplete placental separation, premature rupture of membranes, and miscarriage.[28,29] A recent study by Sago and colleagues[30] reported up to 90% survival of at least 1 fetus after fetoscopic laser surgery. The rate of major neurologic complications in the born babies at 6 months of age was less than 5%. The investigators also noticed a decrease in survival rate in Quintero stages 3 and 4 pregnancies.

Discordant Twin Growth

Discordant twin growth is described as a difference of 20% or more in estimated fetal weights. Discordant growth can occur in monochorionic or dichorionic pregnancies. Discordant growth occurs in 7% to 11% of monochorionic diamniotic twin pregnancies and is an important cause of fetal morbidity and mortality. Discordant growth can occur in combination with TTTS, in isolation, or as the result of anomalies or aneuploidy in 1 of the twins. Lewi and colleagues[31] described unequal placental sharing as the cause of isolated early onset discordant growth appearing by 20 weeks of gestation. The placentas in these pregnancies were more unequally shared and had larger arterioarterial anastomoses as well as larger total anastomotic diameter. The discordant growth was apparent from first trimester or at 16 weeks in most of their study subjects. Most of these subjects also had abnormal umbilical artery Doppler findings. Twin gestations with late onset discordant growth appearing after 26 weeks of gestation demonstrated an intertwin transfusion imbalance. Interestingly, most of these study subjects demonstrated severe intertwin hemoglobin level differences at birth.[31]

Because of its size, the smaller twin produces less urine than the larger twin. In severe cases, the smaller twin may develop oligohydramnios or anhydramnios. Isolated discordant growth can be diagnosed if there is no evidence of polyhydramnios in the larger twin, and it is less likely to result in developmental delays than TTTS.

Characterization of umbilical artery flow pattern in the smaller twin is suggested as a classification method of discordant growth in twin pregnancies. In monochorionic pregnancies, umbilical artery Doppler waveform reflects downstream placental vascular resistance and blood flow across the anastomoses.[29]

Gratacós and colleagues[32] classified monochorionic twins with selective intrauterine growth restriction at 18 to 26 weeks into 3 types. Type 1 included those twins with normal umbilical artery Doppler waveform in the smaller twin. This group

had mild unequal placental sharing with large artery-to-artery anastomoses. Outcome for this group was generally good. Type 2 included those with absent or reversed end diastolic flow in the smaller twin. This group behaved similar to growth-restricted singleton pregnancies. In this group, Doppler evaluation of ductus venosus was necessary. An absent or reversed a wave in the ductus venosus usually indicated imminent fetal demise. The fetal placenta was also more unequally shared but did not show any large artery-to-artery anastomoses. This group had the worse prognosis, and 90% eventually showed signs of deterioration and imminent demise. Type 3 included those with intermittently absent or reversed end diastolic flow in the umbilical artery in the smaller twin. This pattern was most commonly seen in the early onset discordant growth and was accompanied by a large artery-to-artery anastomosis and gross unequal placental sharing. This group had an intermediate prognosis but was also the most unpredictable. Unexpected fetal demise without any signs of deterioration occurred in about 15% of cases and half of those involved both twins.[32]

Ultrasonographic examination plays an important role in the management of discordant twin growth. Factors that affect clinical decision making include fluid volume, Doppler parameters, fetal nonstress test, and biophysical profile. Also, in selective cases with severe complications, ultrasound-guided feticide of the smaller twin can be offered as an option to improve survival of the larger twin.

Twin Anemia-Polycythemia Sequence

This entity is described in monochorionic twin gestations with discordant hemoglobin levels. One twin is larger, with polycythemia and plethora at birth, whereas the other twin is smaller with anemia at birth. Twin anemia-polycythemia sequence (TAPS) can occur spontaneously in previously uncomplicated pregnancies or after an incomplete laser surgery for TTTS. TAPS is also seen in late onset isolated discordant twin growth. The placentas of twins with TAPS show few small unidirectional artery-to-vein anastomoses without compensating artery-to-artery anastomosis suggesting that TAPS is the result of a chronic net transfusion across the small anastomoses.[33]

Doppler ultrasonography of the middle cerebral artery (MCA) is used to diagnose TAPS. The diagnostic criteria include peak systolic velocity of the MCA greater than 1.5 multiples of the median in 1 twin, suggesting anemia, and MCA peak systolic velocity less than 0.8 multiples of the median in the other twin, suggesting polycythemia. The diagnosis of TAPS can be considered only if TTTS is absent. TTTS can be excluded by ultrasonographic evaluation that would demonstrate mild discordance of the amniotic fluid, which would not comply with the criteria of TTTS.[34]

Twin Reversed Arterial Pattern

Twin reversed arterial pattern (TRAP) is a rare complication unique to monochorionic pregnancies, with an occurrence rate of 0.3%.[35] TRAP is characterized by the lack of formation of a defined cardiac structure in 1 twin (acardiac twin), who is then hemodynamically dependent on the other twin (pump twin). There are artery-to-artery anastomoses within the placental mass, and the acardiac twin is perfused with deoxygenated blood from the pump twin. This process results in reversed perfusion in the acardiac twin because blood enters the fetus via the umbilical artery. The acardiac twin's condition is incompatible with survival, whereas the pump twin's condition has variable prognosis. The pump twin is at risk for fetal hydrops due to high cardiac output and polyhydramnios. There is an increased risk of premature labor in TRAP as well.[35]

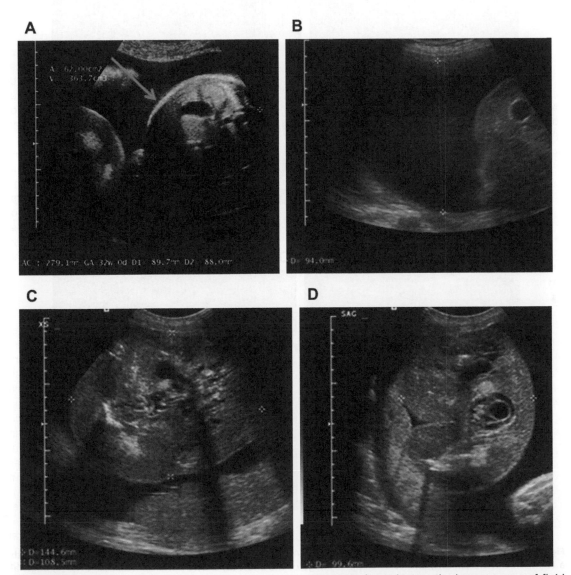

Fig. 10. TRAP sequence. (A) Normal growth is seen in the pump twin (arrow). Note the large amount of fluid surrounding the pump twin (B), compatible with polyhydramnios. (C, D) Acardiac twin appears deformed with only the torso and 1 developed leg. Note the significant soft tissue edema.

Ultrasonography plays an important role in the assessment of TRAP pregnancies. The sonographic findings in the acardiac twin include absence of a cardiac structure, often no identifiable cranial structure, variable presence and appearance of the upper extremities, recognizable torso, and presence of lower extremities, which can move spontaneously (**Fig. 10**).[35] Doppler ultrasonography is very useful for confirmation of this diagnosis. There is a high incidence of the presence of a single umbilical artery in the acardiac twin, which would demonstrate reversed flow on Doppler evaluation. Doppler ultrasonography is used to assess the pump twin for signs of impending fetal hydrops. These signs include reversed flow in the ductus venosus, reversed flow in the inferior vena cava, and pulsatile flow in the umbilical vein. Fetal echocardiography should be considered for the pump twin once the diagnosis of TRAP is established. Myocardial

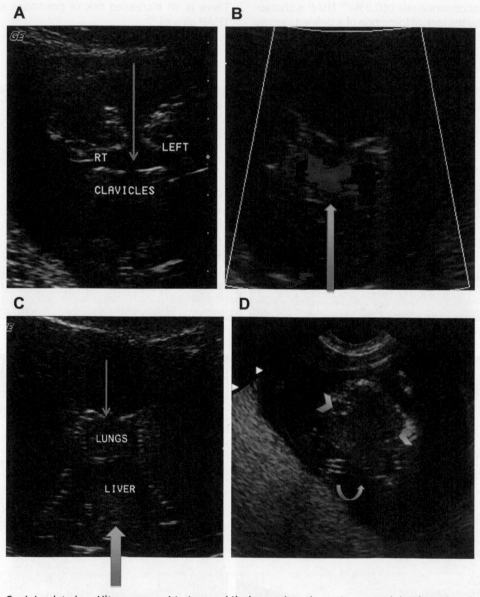

Fig. 11. Conjoined twins. Ultrasonographic image (*A*) shows that the twins were joined at the chest with a common clavicle (*arrow*), and color Doppler image of the chest (*B*) shows a shared heart (*arrow*). (*C*) Sagittal ultrasonographic image shows shared lungs (*small arrow*) and shared liver (*large arrow*). (*D*) Transverse image at the level of the cord insertion shows 2 separate stomachs (*arrowheads*) and a single cord insertion (*curved arrowhead*). RT, right.

thickening and tricuspid regurgitation should raise suspicion for high-output cardiac failure. Doppler ultrasonography can also demonstrate the location of arterial anastomoses on the surface of the placenta.[36,37] Schwärzler and colleagues[38] reported the ability to diagnose TRAP by transvaginal ultrasonography in as early as 12 weeks of gestation. More recently, Bonilla-Musoles and colleagues[37] reported a case series, in which 3D sonography assisted in confirming the diagnosis of TRAP and assisted in determining the extent of structural anomalies in the acardiac twin.

Untreated TRAP pregnancies have a mortality rate of 50% to 75%.[35] The size of the acardiac fetus is the most important prognostic factor and may be detected before development of signs of cardiac failure in the pump twin. Moore and colleagues[39] calculated the ratio of fetal weights between the acardiac twin and its pump twin in 49 TRAP pregnancies. They reported increased incidence rates of preterm labor, polyhydramnios, and heart failure when the weight ratio was more than 70%. In addition, rapid growth of the acardiac twin is associated with a poor prognosis.[39] Sonographic fetal weight measurement by routine fetal biometry could be difficult because of the amorphous structure of the acardiac twin.[40]

Recently, Wong and Sepulveda[35] suggested using the abdominal circumference ratio as a prognostic factor in evaluating the effect of the acardiac twin on the pump twin. They suggested that an abdominal circumference ratio of more than 50% should be regarded as a negative prognostic factor and should prompt intervention. Bornstein and colleagues[40] suggested in a case report that 3D volume calculation of the fetal body can be used to estimate the fetal size. They emphasize that such calculations can be obtained rapidly and easily without any specific organ estimation and therefore does not depend on the morphology of the acardiac fetus. Dashe and colleagues[41] reported on the utility of Doppler imaging of the fetal umbilical artery in predicting the outcome in TRAP pregnancies. In their study they measured the resistive indices of the umbilical arteries and found that larger differences between the resistive indices are associated with improved outcome of the pump twin, whereas smaller resistive index differences were associated with poor outcome of the pump twin, including cardiac failure and CNS hypoperfusion.

Conservative management of TRAP pregnancies is suggested by some investigators if the acardiac twin is smaller than the pump twin, there are no signs of cardiac failure in the pump twin, and there is no evidence of polyhydramnios. Once intervention is considered, treatment usually involves termination of the acardiac twin to improve survival of the pump twin. Timely intervention can improve the pump twin's survival by 76%. Ultrasonography can be used for guidance of invasive techniques such as ligation of the acardiac umbilical cord after 24 weeks, radiofrequency ablation of acardiac umbilical artery, or fetoscopic laser coagulation of shunt vessels at less than 24 weeks' gestation.[42,43]

Intrauterine Fetal Growth Restriction

The incidence of intrauterine fetal growth restriction (IUGR) in twin pregnancies is approximately 15% to 25%. In a recent study Fox and colleagues[44] investigated the association of maternal risk factors with intrauterine growth restriction in twin pregnancies. They defined IUGR as a fetal weight of less than 10th percentile for gestational age, a birth weight of less than 5th percentile, or birth weight discordant growth of 20% or more. The investigators found no significant association between twin IUGR and any maternal risk factors such as maternal age, weight, in vitro fertilization, hypertension, diabetes, thrombophilia, or pregnancy reduction. The higher rates of IUGR in twin pregnancies may account for some of the increased risk of intrauterine fetal death, neonatal mortality, and cerebral palsy than in singleton pregnancies.[45,46] Recent studies have shown that IUGR is associated with a late-life increased prevalence of metabolic syndrome, a condition associating obesity with hypertension; type 2 diabetes mellitus; and cardiovascular disease.[47] All twin pregnancies should be closely monitored for development of IUGR by serial ultrasonographic examinations.

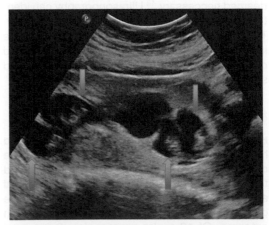

Fig. 12. Septuplets (7 fetuses) in a patient who underwent in vitro fertilization. Multiple gestational sacs are noted within the uterine cavity (4 fetuses/sacs are noted in this image, *arrows*).

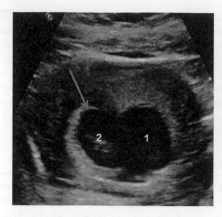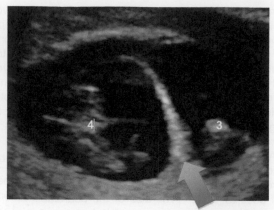

Fig. 13. In septuplets, chorionicity and amnionicity follow the same rules as in twins. In this example, fetuses 1 and 2 are monochorionic diamniotic (note thin membrane, *small arrow*), whereas fetuses 3 and 4 are dichorionic diamniotic (note thick membrane, *large arrow*).

Conjoined Twins

This condition results from fusion of twins of variable degree and at variable sites. Conjoined twins continue to raise significant ethical and legal dilemmas. There are many issues, such as authority of consent, accepted operative risks, and postoperative quality of life, that still remain to be universally decided upon. Accurate prenatal diagnosis of complex anatomic connections and associated anomalies play an imperative role in counseling parents as well as planning potential postnatal surgical separation. Detailed diagnosis of complex anatomic connections and any associated anomalies has been possible only recently with the advent of advanced ultrasonographic techniques, fetal magnetic resonance imaging, and fetal echocardiography. These examinations can also help in planning ex utero intrapartum treatment procedure if emergent separation is deemed neccessary.[48] Ultrasonography can identify conjoined twins as early as in the first trimester. The best indicator of this diagnosis is twins that are inseparable (**Fig. 11**). Close examination would demonstrate contiguous skin covering the joined sites.

MULTIPLE GESTATIONS BEYOND TWINS

Between 1973 and 1990, the rate of triplets and higher-order births increased at 7 times the rate of singletons.[1] The increased rates are attributed to several factors including advanced maternal age and advanced infertility treatments. Multiple gestations are at higher risk for poor birth outcome. Of 10 triplet pregnancies, 9 are born preterm with an average birth weight that is half of that of a singleton birth. The infant death rate for triplets and higher-order pregnancies are 12

times higher than that in a singleton pregnancy.[49] Higher orders of multiple gestations may share chorionic and amniotic sacs. Careful ultrasonographic examination is crucial in determination of the relationship of the fetuses to each other (**Figs. 12** and **13**). The chorionicity and amnionicity of each fetus is determined using the same guidelines for twin pregnancies. Each fetus carries the same perinatal risk factors of its corresponding category of chorionicity and amnionicity and would require serial evaluations accordingly. Ultrasonographic examinations are performed to assess fetal anatomic structures, possible anomalies, and complications. Serial examinations are used to monitor fetal growth. Ultrasonography can also assist in reduction of the number of fetuses, if desired by the parents.

REFERENCES

1. Luke B. The changing pattern of multiple births in the United States: maternal and infant characteristics, 1973 and 1990. Obstet Gynecol 1994;84:101–6.
2. Aston KI, Peterson CM, Carrell DT. Monozygotic twinning associated with assisted reproductive technologies: a review. Reproduction 2008;136:377–86.
3. The 2010 statistical abstract: births, deaths, marriages and divorces. Washington, DC: U.S. Census Bureau; 2010.
4. Galan H, Pandipati S, Filly R. Ultrasound evaluation of fetal biometry and normal and abnormal fetal growth. In: Callen P, editor. Ultrasonography in obstetrics and gynecology. 4th edition. Philadelphia: W.B. Saunders Company; 2000. p. 225–65.
5. Mahony BS, Filly RA, Callen PW. Amnionicity and chorionicity in twin pregnancies: prediction using ultrasound. Radiology 1985;155:205–9.

6. Sadler T. Langman's medical embryology. 11th edition. Baltimore (MD): Lippincott Williams & Wilkins; 2010.

7. Hill LM, Chenevey P, Hecker J, et al. Sonographic determination of first trimester twin chorionicity and amnionicity. J Clin Ultrasound 1996;24:305–8.

8. Doubilet PM, Benson CB. "Appearing twin": under-counting of multiple gestations on early first trimester sonograms. J Ultrasound Med 1998;17:199–203; [quiz: 205–6].

9. Trop I. The twin peak sign. Radiology 2001;220:68–9.

10. Bromley B, Benacerraf B. Using the number of yolk sacs to determine amnionicity in early first trimester monochorionic twins. J Ultrasound Med 1995;14: 415–9.

11. Townsend RR, Simpson GF, Filly RA. Membrane thickness in ultrasound prediction of chorionicity of twin gestations. J Ultrasound Med 1988;7: 327–32.

12. Sherer DM. Adverse perinatal outcome of twin pregnancies according to chorionicity: review of the literature. Am J Perinatol 2001;18:23–37.

13. Lewi L, Gucciardo L, Van Mieghem T, et al. Monochorionic diamniotic twin pregnancies: natural history and risk stratification. Fetal Diagn Ther 2010;27:121–33.

14. Gandhi M, Cleary-Goldman J, Ferrara L, et al. The association between vasa previa, multiple gestations, and assisted reproductive technology. Am J Perinatol 2008;25:587–9.

15. Sherer DM, Anyaegbunam A. Prenatal ultrasonographic morphologic assessment of the umbilical cord: a review. Part I. Obstet Gynecol Surv 1997;52: 506–14.

16. Sherer DM, Anyaegbunam A. Prenatal ultrasonographic morphologic assessment of the umbilical cord: a review. Part II. Obstet Gynecol Surv 1997; 52:515–23.

17. Henrich W, Tutschek B. Cord entanglement in monoamniotic twins: 2D and 3D colour Doppler studies. Ultraschall Med 2008;29(Suppl 5):271–2.

18. Dias T, Mahsud-Dornan S, Bhide A, et al. Cord entanglement and perinatal outcome in monoamniotic twin pregnancies. Ultrasound Obstet Gynecol 2010;35:201–4.

19. Magann EF, Chauhan SP, Whitworth NS, et al. The accuracy of the summated amniotic fluid index in evaluating amniotic fluid volume in twin pregnancies. Am J Obstet Gynecol 1997;177:1041–5.

20. Lewi L. Cord entanglement in monoamniotic twins: does it really matter? Ultrasound Obstet Gynecol 2010;35:139–41.

21. Jain V, Fisk NM. The twin-twin transfusion syndrome. Clin Obstet Gynecol 2004;47:181–202.

22. Quintero RA, Morales WJ, Allen MH, et al. Staging of twin-twin transfusion syndrome. J Perinatol 1999;19: 550–5.

23. Sueters M, Middeldorp JM, Lopriore E, et al. Timely diagnosis of twin-to-twin transfusion syndrome in monochorionic twin pregnancies by biweekly sonography combined with patient instruction to report onset of symptoms. Ultrasound Obstet Gynecol 2006;28:659–64.

24. Sebire NJ, D'Ercole C, Hughes K, et al. Increased nuchal translucency thickness at 10–14 weeks of gestation as a predictor of severe twin-to-twin transfusion syndrome. Ultrasound Obstet Gynecol 1997; 10:86–9.

25. Lewi L, Lewi P, Diemert A, et al. The role of ultrasound examination in the first trimester and at 16 weeks' gestation to predict fetal complications in monochorionic diamniotic twin pregnancies. Am J Obstet Gynecol 2008;199:493, e1–7.

26. Senat MV, Deprest J, Boulvain M, et al. Endoscopic laser surgery versus serial amnioreduction for severe twin-to-twin transfusion syndrome. N Engl J Med 2004;351:136–44.

27. Graef C, Ellenrieder B, Hecher K, et al. Long-term neurodevelopmental outcome of 167 children after intrauterine laser treatment for severe twin-twin transfusion syndrome. Am J Obstet Gynecol 2006; 194:303–8.

28. Cavicchioni O, Yamamoto M, Robyr R, et al. Intrauterine fetal demise following laser treatment in twin-to-twin transfusion syndrome. BJOG 2006;113: 590–4.

29. Yamamoto M, El Murr L, Robyr R, et al. Incidence and impact of perioperative complications in 175 fetoscopy-guided laser coagulations of chorionic plate anastomoses in fetofetal transfusion syndrome before 26 weeks of gestation. Am J Obstet Gynecol 2005;193:1110–6.

30. Sago H, Hayashi S, Saito M, et al. The outcome and prognostic factors of twin-twin transfusion syndrome following fetoscopic laser surgery. Prenat Diagn 2010;30:1185–91.

31. Lewi L, Gucciardo L, Huber A, et al. Clinical outcome and placental characteristics of monochorionic diamniotic twin pairs with early- and late-onset discordant growth. Am J Obstet Gynecol 2008;199: 511, e1–7.

32. Gratacós E, Lewi L, Muñoz B, et al. A classification system for selective intrauterine growth restriction in monochorionic pregnancies according to umbilical artery Doppler flow in the smaller twin. Ultrasound Obstet Gynecol 2007;30:28–34.

33. Lopriore E, Deprest J, Slaghekke F, et al. Placental characteristics in monochorionic twins with and without twin anemia-polycythemia sequence. Obstet Gynecol 2008;112:753–8.

34. Lewi L. Monochorionic diamniotic twin pregnancies pregnancy outcome, risk stratification and lessons learnt from placental examination. Verh K Acad Geneeskd Belg 2010;72:5–15.

35. Wong AE, Sepulveda W. Acardiac anomaly: current issues in prenatal assessment and treatment. Prenat Diagn 2005;25:796–806.

36. Van Allen MI, Smith DW, Shepard TH. Twin reversed arterial perfusion (TRAP) sequence: a study of 14 twin pregnancies with acardius. Semin Perinatol 1983;7:285–93.

37. Bonilla-Musoles F, Machado LE, Raga F, et al. Fetus acardius: two- and three-dimensional ultrasonographic diagnoses. J Ultrasound Med 2001;20: 1117–27.

38. Schwärzler P, Ville Y, Moscosco G, et al. Diagnosis of twin reversed arterial perfusion sequence in the first trimester by transvaginal color Doppler ultrasound. Ultrasound Obstet Gynecol 1999;13:143–6.

39. Moore TR, Gale S, Benirschke K. Perinatal outcome of forty-nine pregnancies complicated by acardiac twinning. Am J Obstet Gynecol 1990;163:907–12.

40. Bornstein E, Monteagudo A, Dong R, et al. Detection of twin reversed arterial perfusion sequence at the time of first-trimester screening: the added value of 3-dimensional volume and color Doppler sonography. J Ultrasound Med 2008;27:1105–9.

41. Dashe JS, Fernandez CO, Twickler DM. Utility of Doppler velocimetry in predicting outcome in twin reversed-arterial perfusion sequence. Am J Obstet Gynecol 2001;185:135–9.

42. Hirose M, Murata A, Kita N, et al. Successful intra-uterine treatment with radiofrequency ablation in a case of acardiac twin pregnancy complicated with a hydropic pump twin. Ultrasound Obstet Gynecol 2004;23:509–12.

43. Tan TY, Sepulveda W. Acardiac twin: a systematic review of minimally invasive treatment modalities. Ultrasound Obstet Gynecol 2003;22:409–19.

44. Fox NS, Rebarber A, Klauser CK, et al. Intrauterine growth restriction in twin pregnancies: incidence and associated risk factors. Am J Perinatol 2010. [Epub ahead of print].

45. Demissie K, Ananth CV, Martin J, et al. Fetal and neonatal mortality among twin gestations in the United States: the role of intrapair birth weight discordance. Obstet Gynecol 2002;100:474–80.

46. Salihu HM, Garces IC, Sharma PP, et al. Stillbirth and infant mortality among Hispanic singletons, twins, and triplets in the United States. Obstet Gynecol 2005;106:789–96.

47. Valsamakis G, Kanaka-Gantenbein C, Malamitsi-Puchner A, et al. Causes of intrauterine growth restriction and the postnatal development of the metabolic syndrome. Ann N Y Acad Sci 2006; 1092:138–47.

48. Mackenzie TC, Crombleholme TM, Johnson MP, et al. The natural history of prenatally diagnosed conjoined twins. J Pediatr Surg 2002;37:303–9.

49. Keith L, Breborowicz G. Triplet pregnancies and their aftermaths. Part I: basic considerations. Int J Fertil Womens Med 2002;47:254–64.

Complex Deliveries in Obstetrics

Edith Y. Cheng, MD, MS[a,b],*

KEYWORDS

- Cesearean delivery • Ex utero intrapartum therapy
- EXIT • Placenta previa

Obstetricians have the unique responsibility of caring for 2 patients, the mother and her fetus, simultaneously. Most healthy mothers have an uncomplicated pregnancy and give birth to a healthy baby. However, there are situations in which competing goals for outcomes between the mother and the fetus compromise the mother to save the baby or generate permanent morbidity to the child to protect the life of the mother (and the child). This article discusses 2 perinatal conditions that illustrate the complexity of the maternal and fetal relationship at delivery and the importance of multidisciplinary cooperation in enhancing successful outcomes for both mother and baby.

MANAGEMENT STRATEGIES FOR ABNORMAL PLACENTATION
Background

Abnormalities of placentation can cause significant maternal, fetal, and neonatal morbidity and mortality. The severity of abnormal placental attachment is defined by the depth of invasion of the chorionic villi: (1) accreta, in which chorionic villi invade into the myometrium rather than being restricted within the decidual basalis; (2) increta, in which chorionic villi invade into but not through the full thickness of the myometrium; and (3) percreta, in which chorionic villi invade through the myometrium. Placenta accreta is the most common histologic finding in hysterectomy specimens, accounting for approximately 82% of cases; increta is found in 12% and percreta in

6%.[1] Because of the abnormal tissue attachment, labor and delivery with placenta accreta (increta and percreta) are associated with hemorrhage when complete detachment of the placenta is not successful. Life-threatening complications include transfusion with large amount of blood products, emergency laparotomy, and hysterectomy leading to comorbidities such as cystotomy, ureteral damage, damage to the bowel and adjacent pelvic structures, coagulopathy, transfusion-associated lung injury, acute respiratory distress, and postoperative infection and fistula formation. A maternal mortality rate as high as 7% has been reported for placenta accreta.[2]

The incidence of placenta accreta has increased from 0.8 per 1000 deliveries in the 1980s to 3 per 1000 deliveries in the past decade because of the changing maternal demographics and obstetric practice patterns.[3–6] Risk factors for placenta accreta include high parity, advanced maternal age, previous uterine surgery, and specifically, previous cesarean delivery with placenta previa. In fact, in the absence of placenta previa, the risk for placenta accreta is 0.03% after 1 previous cesarean delivery and less than 1% for up to 5 cesarean deliveries.[6] At 6 or more cesarean deliveries, the risk for placenta accreta is 4.7%. However, if placenta previa is present, the risk of placenta accreta is 3% after the first cesarean delivery and is as high as 40% or more after the third cesarean delivery (**Table 1**). Both posterior and anterior placenta previa are at an increased risk for placenta accreta, and the risk is increased

a Division of Maternal Fetal Medicine, Department of Obstetrics and Gynecology, University of Washington, 1959 NE Pacific Street, Box 356460, Seattle, WA 98195, USA
b Division of Medical Genetics, Department of Internal Medicine, University of Washington, Seattle, WA 98195, USA
* Division of Maternal Fetal Medicine, Department of Obstetrics and Gynecology, University of Washington, 1959 NE Pacific Street, Box 356460, Seattle, WA 98195.
E-mail address: chengels@u.washington.edu

Ultrasound Clin 6 (2011) 133–141
doi:10.1016/j.cult.2011.02.004

Table 1
Observed frequency of placenta accreta as a function of the number of cesarean deliveries and absence or presence of coexisting placenta previa

Number of Cesarean Deliveries	Frequency of Placenta Accreta (%)	
	With Placenta Previa	Without Placenta Previa
1	3.3	0.03
2	11	0.2
3	40	0.1
4	61	0.8
5	67	0.8
6	67	4.7

Placenta previa and a history of cesarean delivery are the most significant risk factors for placenta accreta.

Data from Silver RM, Landon MB, Rouse DJ, et al. Maternal morbidity associated with multiple repeat cesarean deliveries. Obstet Gynecol 2006;107:1226–32.

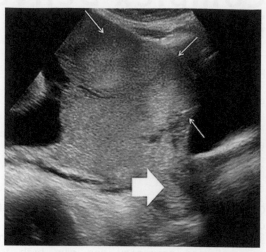

Fig. 1. Sagittal ultrasonographic image of the cervix (*large arrow*) showing the presence of placenta previa with invasion (*arrows*). Bladder wall does not appear to be invaded.

substantially if there is placental tissue at the location of the uterine scar.[7]

Prenatal Detection of Abnormal Placentation—Role of Imaging

Ultrasonography

Early detection of abnormal placental attachment would be of great benefit for preoperative planning and counseling. Historically, placenta accreta/percreta were rarely diagnosed in the first trimester. However, with the increase in cesarean deliveries and the use of first-trimester ultrasonography, case reports of first-trimester placenta accreta, percreta with infiltration, and extrusion of gestational *sac* through the lower uterine scar are now appearing in the literature with higher frequency, and the characteristics of placenta accreta/percreta in early gestation are now being evaluated.[8–10] However, in spite of the rapidly improving ultrasonography technology and increasing use of first-trimester ultrasonography in prenatal screening, the ultrasonographic characteristics of placenta accreta in the first trimester have not been well established and the predictive value of first-trimester ultrasonography for the diagnosis of placenta accreta has not been systematically investigated.

Second-trimester transabdominal gray-scale ultrasonography and 2-dimensional color Doppler are the simplest and most commonly used methods for the evaluation of placental attachment to the myometrium (**Fig. 1**). The combination of a low-lying placenta or placenta previa and a history of at least 1 cesarean delivery remains the most important diagnostic predictor of placenta accreta.[6] Thus, inquiring about the patient's obstetric history is a recommended practice. With this information, high-risk patients should have a targeted evaluation of the anterior myometrial-placental interface and the myometrial–bladder wall interface. In a prospective study of 34 women with placenta previa and a history of cesarean delivery, Finberg and Williams[11] were the first to describe specific ultrasonographic criteria for the diagnosis of abnormal placentation. The 3 diagnostic criteria include (1) loss of the hypoechoic retroplacental zone, (2) thinning of the hyperechoic uterine serosa–bladder interface, and (3) presence of focal exophytic masses. The use of these criteria in high-risk women resulted in a sensitivity of 93% and a specificity of 73% to diagnose or exclude placenta accreta, respectively. Comstock and colleagues[12] evaluated the sensitivity and specificity of each specific criteria associated with placenta accreta in women undergoing second-trimester ultrasonography. The 3 criteria evaluated in their study were (1) the obliteration of the clear space between the uterus and placenta; (2) visualization of placental lacunae, defined as multiple, linear, irregular vascular spaces within the placenta that are often referred to as a "Swiss cheese" or "moth eaten" appearance of the placenta; and (3) interruption of the posterior bladder wall–uterine interface. In the second trimester, visualization of the placental lacunae had the highest sensitivity to detect placenta accreta (78.6%). Obliteration of the clear space had a sensitivity of 57%, and interruption of the posterior bladder wall–uterine interface had a sensitivity of 21.4%. The sensitivity was 86% with any 1 finding and 89% if 2 or more findings were identified. Moreover, the presence of 2 or more features increased the positive predictive value from 63% to 89%. Twickler and colleagues[13] found that the combination of myometrial thinning of 1 mm or less and large placental lacunae had a high positive predictive value of 72%. The significance of placental lakes in predicting placenta accreta is further supported by Sumigama and colleagues,[14] who identified this feature in 82.4% (14 of 17) women with placenta accreta. Wong and colleagues[1] reported that among 6 sonographic criteria, vessels crossing interface disruption sites, disruption of the placental–uterine wall interface, and vessels bridging from the placenta to the uterine margin had the highest likelihood ratios (42.9, 25.3, and 18.4, respectively) for placenta accreta. **Box 1** summarizes some of the sonographic findings associated with placenta accreta.

Magnetic resonance imaging
There has been long-standing interest in the role of magnetic resonance imaging (MRI) in the diagnosis of placenta previa (**Fig. 2**). Small retrospective reviews and case studies have suggested improved detection of placenta accreta using MRI, but some of these reports did not have comparisons with ultrasonography, pathologic confirmation, or controls, and none of them had defined MRI characteristics for placenta accreta.[15–20] Kim and Narra[19] were the first to define the appearance of the placental-myometrial interface as having 3 layers of differing signal intensity, with the inner layer having a low signal intensity; middle layer, high intensity; and outer layer, low signal intensity. In placenta accreta, focal nonvisualization of the inner layer was observed. However, in this study, the radiology reviewer was not blinded to the diagnosis or the location of the placenta accreta as visualized by ultrasonography. The criteria used by Lam and

---

Box 1
Second-trimester sonographic findings associated with placenta accreta

Loss of hypoechoic retroplacental space

Retroplacental myometrial thinning of 1 mm or less

Placental lacunae (lakes)

Bridging blood vessels or placental tissue across

    Uterine to placental margin

    Myometrial-bladder interface

    Crossing uterine serosa

---

colleagues[18] include attenuation or nonvisualization of the uterine wall in the area of the placenta, interruption of the tissue plane between the myometrium and bladder wall, and overt invasion of the myometrium by the placenta. Although the criteria seemed reasonable, there were 5 false-negative results in their study and no control subjects.

Palacios Jaraquemada and Bruno[21] investigated the correlation between MRI-provided topographic information and the depth of placental invasion in 300 women with ultrasonographic findings of placenta accreta with the findings obtained during surgery and/or pathologic examination. MRI modified the depth of invasion in 90 patients, diagnosed previously unsuspected parametrial extension in 11, and reclassified 11 others as having placenta previa without accreta. There were 4 false-positive cases, predominantly because of the artifact created by thick vessels in the bladder-myometrial interface that gave the diagnostic impression of placenta percreta. There were 3 false-negative cases because of studies with incomplete sequences. However, these patients were surgically approached as having placenta accreta/percreta based on the high-risk clinical history and ultrasonographic findings. Although there were no controls in this study, the findings would suggest that MRI has an added benefit in allowing the obstetrician to determine the timing of delivery and adopt the surgical approach; the former has a significant effect on neonatal and long-term morbidity for the child, and the latter requires precise surgical planning, including the type of incision, transfusion support, and vascular control to potentially decrease maternal morbidity.

The first blinded study on the use of prenatal MRI to predict placenta accreta, increta, or percreta was conducted by Lax and colleagues.[22] In this retrospective study, the placental MRI characteristics of 10 patients with pathologically confirmed placental invasion were compared with 10 patients without placental abnormality. Of 7 characteristics on which the 2 blinded experts were to score, 3 features of MRI in patients with placental invasion seemed to be useful for diagnosis: uterine bulging, heterogeneous signal intensity within the placenta, and presence of dark intraplacental bands on T2-weighted imaging. Similar results were subsequently reported by Teo and colleagues.[23]

Studies comparing the sensitivities and specificities of prenatal ultrasonography and prenatal MRI for the diagnosis of placenta accreta have yielded conflicting results.[24,25] In a study by Warshak and colleagues,[24] among 39 high-risk women with pathologically confirmed placenta accreta, ultrasonography predicted placenta accreta in 30 (sensitivity, 77%), and in 414 women without placenta

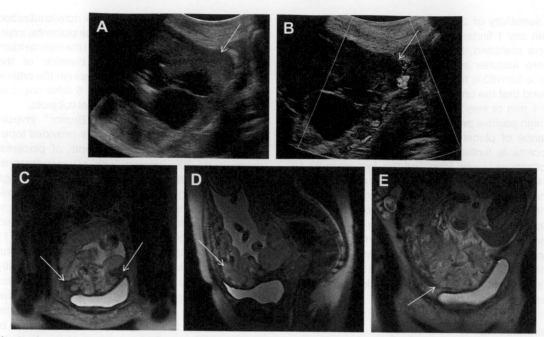

Fig. 2. Placenta percreta. Sagittal ultrasonographic image (A) and color Doppler image (B) of the lower uterine segment show extension of the placenta outside the uterine wall (*arrow*) with increased vascularity, which is consistent with placenta percreta. (C–E) MRI performed to map the location and extension of the invasion shows complete loss of integrity of the uterine wall (*arrows*) with extension of the placenta outside the uterus, which was consistent with placenta percreta on surgery.

previa, it excluded placenta accreta in 398 (specificity, 96%). A total of 42 women underwent MRI because of inconclusive ultrasonographic findings. MRI accurately predicted placenta accreta in 23 of 26 cases (sensitivity, 88%) and correctly excluded placenta accreta in all 14 cases (specificity, 100%). In 32 high-risk women, Dwyer and colleagues[25] reported a higher sensitivity (93%) but a lower specificity (71%) for ultrasonography in the prenatal diagnosis and prenatal exclusion of placenta accreta, respectively, whereas for MRI, the sensitivity was 80% (12 of 15) and the specificity was 65% (11 of 17), respectively. Ultrasonographic and MRI findings were discordant in 7 of 32 women, with ultrasonography being correct in 5 and MRI correct in 2. It is reasonable to conclude that at present, evidence supporting the routine use of MRI for the prenatal diagnosis of placenta accreta in high-risk women is lacking. However, MRI may be helpful as an adjunct in high-risk cases in which the ultrasonographic features are inconclusive.

Management of Placenta Accreta/Increta/Percreta

The immediate intrapartum complication of placenta accreta is uncontrollable hemorrhage requiring hysterectomy. Thus, it is intuitively logical

to hypothesize that antenatal diagnosis would facilitate counseling, timing of delivery, and preparation to ensure a safe delivery of the fetus, as well as limit the maternal comorbidities of an emergent postpartum or cesarean hysterectomy. The optimal timing for a planned delivery and surgical approach are controversial; it is a compromise between minimizing the risk of morbidity related to late preterm prematurity and the risk of significant maternal morbidity or mortality. Eller and colleagues[26] reported a mean gestational age of 32.2 weeks for emergency deliveries among patients with antenatally suspected placenta accreta. O'Brien and colleagues[2] reported that after 35 weeks, 93% of patients with placenta accreta had hemorrhage and required emergent delivery. Among 8 maternal deaths, 4 occurred in women who delivered after 36 weeks of gestation. Eller and colleagues[26] further reported that among 15 of 57 women with an antenatal diagnosis of placenta accreta, in whom an attempt was made to remove the placenta, all required immediate hysterectomy because of massive hemorrhage. They concluded that the most influential variable on maternal outcome was whether an attempt was made to remove the placenta. Intraoperative blood loss among women undergoing cesarean hysterectomy for placenta accreta typically ranges from 2 to 5 L. Prenatal detection and planned cesarean hysterectomy has been reported to decrease blood loss.[27]

Other preoperative strategies to minimize maternal complications include presurgical placement of ureteral stents,[26] preoperative pelvic artery embolization,[28,29] and staged delayed delivery after selective embolization of uterine and placental bed at the time of delivery.[30] None of these additional preoperative approaches have been evaluated in large studies; therefore, their role as part of the surgical preparation for planned cesarean hysterectomy needs further evaluation.

The ideal time for delivery is equally controversial because there is little evidence to guide physicians in their choice of the optimal gestational age for delivery. The benefits of a scheduled delivery to minimize maternal morbidity are juxtaposed against exposure of the neonate to complications of prematurity. The risk of hemorrhage increases with gestational age, with more than 90% of women with placenta previa/accreta having symptomatic bleeding before 37 weeks of gestation. Warshak and colleagues[27] observed that only 9 of 62 patients with a predelivery diagnosis delivered after 36 weeks and 4 of them required emergency deliveries for hemorrhage. Robinson and Grobman[31] compared multiple strategies for delivery timing in women with placenta previa/accreta and found that delivery at 34 weeks had the best long-term and short-term outcomes for mother and baby. The study further identified that in women who are not delivered by 36 weeks, amniocentesis for determination of fetal pulmonary maturity did not improve outcome.

In the setting of maternal placenta previa/accreta, the outcome of the neonate is ultimately linked to maternal stability; yet, recent studies have clearly demonstrated that late preterm infants (34 0/7–36 6/7 weeks) experience greater mortality and morbidity than term infants.[32] In the immediate neonatal period, late preterm infants had a higher rate of respiratory distress, infection, and metabolic instability than term infants. More recently, studies identifying increased health care use in the first year of life among late preterm infants have emerged.[33,34] These findings raise at least 2 questions about the long-term health of late preterm infants: one is related to the consequences of prematurity itself and the other is whether the specific therapies and interventions provided to these neonates affect their future health. Thus, the increasing cesarean delivery rates have both an immediate effect on maternal reproductive morbidity and a delayed and perhaps permanent effect on the children delivered under these circumstances.

It seems that there is no ideal strategy for the management of placenta accreta. Predelivery diagnosis provides time for adequate counseling so that all options are discussed and allows the patient to psychologically and emotionally prepare for the surgery, the likelihood of loss of fertility, blood transfusion, and a baby who will be premature and in the intensive care unit. For the surgical team, the surgical approach is planned, and additional preoperative preparations, such as ureteral stents, are considered if, for example, extension into the parametrial space or bladder is suspected based on imaging. Transfusion support, anesthesia, and neonatology are all part of the multidisciplinary cooperation to ensure safe outcomes for mother and baby. At the University of Washington, women with a predelivery diagnosis of placenta previa/accreta who do not desire preservation of fertility are consented for delivery of the infant through a vertical incision high above the placenta. The placenta is left in situ, the uterine incision is rapidly closed for hemostasis, and hysterectomy is completed with the placenta in situ. Although there is a core team to perform most of the planned cases, there is a protocol and checklist that is easily activated for emergent cases. Gestational age at delivery in women who have not had any bleeding is planned for 36 weeks. All pregnancies received a course of betamethasone for acceleration of fetal pulmonary maturity. Amniocentesis for fetal lung maturity is not performed.

EX UTERO INTRAPARTUM THERAPY

Routine prenatal ultrasonographic evaluations of the fetus have resulted in the antenatal identification of fetuses with potential airway compromise. Historically, the unanticipated airway obstruction would result in catastrophic postnatal complications because of the inability to promptly access the newborn's airway. The ex utero intrapartum therapy (EXIT) procedure, originally developed for the reversal of tracheal occlusion at the time of delivery in fetuses who had undergone in utero tracheal occlusion for the treatment of severe congenital diaphragmatic hernia (CDH), has now been adapted and expanded to include any fetal anomaly in which neonatal resuscitation may be compromised.[35] Such anomalies include CDH, large neck, and/or intrathoracic lesions, cardiac lesions, severe micrognathia, and unilateral pulmonary agenesis.[36–41]

The intent of the EXIT procedure is to maintain maternal/placental support of the fetus to provide time for stabilization of the fetus, such as securing the fetal airway, obtaining vascular access, administration of surfactant, surgical resection of masses, and cannulation for extracorporeal membrane oxygenation (ECMO). Preparation for the intrapartum management of these fetuses requires a multidisciplinary assessment in which the benefits of treatment of the fetus are weighed against the risk of maternal complications as a result of prolongation of the intrapartum operative period. Success of the EXIT procedure requires accurate assessment and understanding of the nature of the lesion to coordinate the necessary interventions. In addition, there must be consensus between medical ethicists, radiologists, obstetric anesthesiologists and obstetricians, pediatric surgeons and pediatric anesthesiologists, and neonatologists in the treatment approach and in facilitating parental understanding of the risks and benefits of the proposed procedure to the fetus and mother.

It is the mother who incurs the highest risk during the EXIT procedure while the maternal-fetal bypass state is being established. The foundation for prolongation of placental circulation is uterine relaxation. To achieve uterine relaxation, EXIT procedures are conducted through a cesarean delivery in which the mother undergoes general anesthesia (rather than regional anesthesia as in the case of a routine cesarean delivery). The high concentrations of inhalation agents provide additional uterine relaxation, which is being provided by intravenous infusion of tocolytic agents, usually nitroglycerin. The uterine relaxing agents need to be carefully balanced with fluid administration and vasoactive pressors to maintain maternal hemodynamics and placental perfusion. Given this tenuous balance, adequate

exposure of the uterus, availability of blood products, and the capability to switch to a cesarean hysterectomy are the requirements of an EXIT procedure. Fetal anesthesia is accomplished by the maternal inhalation agents crossing the placental circulation to the fetus. However, because fetal quiescence (of respiration and movements) is critical, intramuscular fetal paralytic agents and narcotics can be directly administered.

The mechanics of the procedure is multilayered, and detailed preparation and checklists of each of the steps are crucial to the safety and success of the procedure. Each group of subspecialty providers has a unique role that is also part of the coordinated collective process in the operating room (**Fig. 3**). At the University of Washington, a diagram of the operating room with placement of equipment, staff, and patient is created and followed each time. Each subspecialty team has a checklist of procedures, and the entire EXIT team meets before the procedure to call out all the intended steps of the case. Transfusion support is notified, and maternal blood products are made available to the team.

The maternal abdominal cavity is usually accessed with a standard Pfannenstiel or low transverse laparotomy incision. However, adequate exposure of the uterus is critical, and a vertical abdominal incision and access should not be overlooked for cosmetic concerns. Access into the uterus is determined by placental location and may necessitate a vertical or even fundal approach if the placenta is anterior. Sterile intraoperative ultrasound guidance can be helpful in mapping the placental edges to determine the hysterotomy

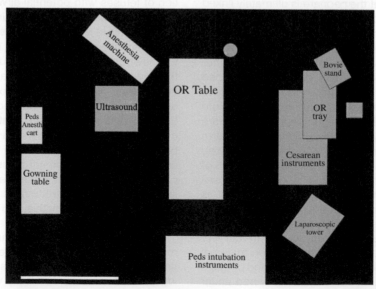

Fig. 3. Layout of the operating room (OR) for an EXIT procedure.

incision and in evaluating the orientation of the fetal head and neck to assist in delivering the head and neck in the optimal orientation for intubation. The hysterotomy incision is first made with a scalpel to a width of only 2 cm. The rest of the incision is extended using a uterine stapling device, which provides hemostasis of the cut myometrial edges.[42]

Fetal procedures are initiated after the fetal head and torso are delivered out of the uterine incision. One provider stabilizes the fetal position while the fetal airway is secured by direct laryngoscopy, bronchoscopy, or tracheostomy (**Fig. 4**). Ultrasonography can be helpful in guidance and confirmation of the intubation. Additional procedures specific to the lesion, such as resection of neck or thoracic masses or cannula placement for ECMO, are performed after the airway is secured. The EXIT procedure and prolongation of uterine relaxation and placental profusion for 2.5 hours have been reported in a case that required dissection of a neck mass.[43] Continuous fetal monitoring is achieved through either the continuous pulse oximeter attached to the fetal hand or continuous ultrasonography with direct visualization or M-mode monitoring. Fetal distress during the procedure can be because of umbilical cord position, uterine volume, and maternal bleeding. A fetal peripheral intravenous line can be placed if necessary.

Just as the EXIT procedure is critical to the health of the fetus, the delivery of the fetus is critical to the safety of the mother. Up to this point, the uterus is maximally relaxed and is at risk for sustained atony and hemorrhage once the placenta is delivered. Thus, coordination between the pediatric/obstetric team and the anesthesia team is crucial so that intravenous oxytocin (Pitocin) administration and reduction of level of inhalation agents occur simultaneously with the clamping of the umbilical cord and delivery of the placenta. The uterine incision is then closed, and the remainder of the operation is completed in the usual fashion for cesarean delivery. Hirose and colleagues[43] found a higher rate of short-term maternal complications among women who underwent EXIT procedures than among women who had routine cesarean delivery, including more wound complications and a higher estimated blood loss (average, 970 mL), but no difference in the length of hospital stay, postpartum hematocrit, or need for transfusion.[44]

The EXIT procedure is now a realistic option for the treatment of fetal conditions in which airway compromise after delivery would otherwise be fatal. In the largest series of 43 fetuses referred to the Center of Fetal Diagnosis and Treatment at The Children's Hospital of Philadelphia from 1996 to 2002, the most common indication was for the management of fetuses with large neck masses or congenital high airway obstruction syndrome.[38] Wagner and Harrison[45] reported that an airway was successfully established in 79% of 29 cases, with an overall survival rate of 69%. Other conditions include large congenital pulmonary adenomatoid malformations or other thoracic/neck masses, unilateral pulmonary agenesis, and CDH. The scope of conditions is now further expanded to craniomaxillofacial anomalies, such as severe congenital micrognathia, as an isolated condition or syndromic as in Cornelia de Lange syndrome.[41]

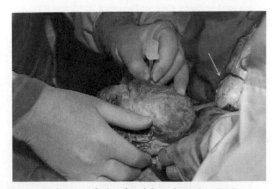

Fig. 4. Delivery of the fetal head in the EXIT procedure, with intubation being performed by the surgeon. Note that the fetal body has not been delivered and the umbilical cord is intact. Note the ultrasound probe (*arrow*) on the maternal abdomen to assess for the appropriate location of the tube in the fetal trachea.

REFERENCES

1. Wong HS, Cheung YK, Zuccollo J, et al. Evaluation of sonographic diagnostic criteria for placenta accreta. J Clin Ultrasound 2008;9:551–9.
2. O'Brien JM, Barton JR, Donaldson ES. Obstetrics: the management of placenta percreta: conservative and operative strategies. Am J Obstet Gynecol 1996;175:1632–8.
3. Flood KM, Said S, Geary M, et al. Changing trends in peripartum hysterectomy over the last 4 decades. Am J Obstet Gynecol 2009;200:632.e1–6.
4. Imudia AN, Awonuga AO, Dbouk T, et al. Incidence, trends, risk factors, indications for and complications associated with cesarean hysterectomy: a 17-year experience from a single institution. Arch Gynecol Obstet 2009;280:619–23.
5. Wu S, Kocherginsky M, Hibbard JU. Abnormal placentation: twenty-year analysis. Am J Obstet Gynecol 2005;192:1458–61.

6. Silver RM, Landon MB, Rouse DJ, et al. Maternal morbidity associated with multiple repeat cesarean deliveries. Obstet Gynecol 2006;107:1226–32.

7. Usta IM, Hobeika EM, Musa AA, et al. Placenta previa-accreta: risk factors and complications. Am J Obstet Gynecol 2005;193:1045–9.

8. Wong HS, Zuccolla J, Tait J, et al. Placenta accreta in the first trimester of pregnancy: sonographic findings. J Clin Ultrasound 2009;37:100–3.

9. Yang JI, Kim HY, Kim HS, et al. Diagnosis in the first trimester of placenta accreta with previous cesarean section. Ultrasound Obstet Gynecol 2009;34:116–8.

10. Comstock CH, Lee W, Vettraino IM, et al. The early sonographic appearance of placenta accreta. J Ultrasound Med 2003;22:12–23.

11. Finberg HJ, Williams JW. Placenta accreta: prospective sonographic diagnosis in patients with placenta previa and prior cesarean section. J Ultrasound Med 1992;11:333–43.

12. Comstock CH, Love JJ, Bronsteen RA, et al. Sonographic detection of placenta accreta in the second and third trimesters of pregnancy. Am J Obstet Gynecol 2004;190:1135–40.

13. Twickler DM, Lucas MJ, Balis AB, et al. Color flow mapping for myometrial invasion in women with a prior cesarean delivery. J Matern Fetal Med 2000;9:330–5.

14. Sumigama S, Itakura A, Ota T, et al. Placenta previa increta/percreta in Japan: a retrospective study of ultrasound findings, management and clinical course. J Obstet Gynaecol Res 2007;33:606–11.

15. Thorp JM, Wells SR, Wiest HH, et al. First-trimester diagnosis of placenta previa percreta by magnetic resonance imaging. Am J Obstet Gynecol 1998;178:616–8.

16. Maldjian D, Adam R, Pelosi M, et al. MRI appearance of placenta percreta and placenta accreta. Magn Reson Imaging 1999;17:965–71.

17. DeFriend DE, Dubbines PA, Hughes PM. Sacculation of the uterus and placenta accreta: MRI appearances. Br J Radiol 2000;73:1323–5.

18. Lam G, Kuller J, MacMahon M. Use of magnetic resonance imaging and ultrasound in the antenatal diagnosis of placenta accreta. J Soc Gynecol Investig 2002;9:37–40.

19. Kim KA, Narra VR. Magnetic resonance imaging with true fast imaging with steady-sate precession and half-Fourier acquisition single-shot turbo spin-echo sequences in cases of suspected placenta accreta. Acta Radiol 2004;45:692–8.

20. Taipale P, Orden MR, Berg M, et al. Prenatal diagnosis of placenta accreta and percreta with ultrasonography, color Doppler, and magnetic resonance imaging. Obstet Gynecol 2004;104:537–40.

21. Palacios Jaraquemada JM, Bruno CH. Magnetic resonance imaging in 300 cases of placenta accreta: surgical correlation of new findings. Acta Obstet Gynecol Scand 2005;84:716–24.

22. Lax A, Prince MR, Mennitt KW, et al. The value of specific MRI features in the evaluation of suspected placental invasion. Magn Reson Imaging 2007;25:87–93.

23. Teo TH, Law YM, Tay KH, et al. Use of magnetic resonance imaging in evaluation of placental invasion. Clin Radiol 2009;64:511–6.

24. Warshak CR, Eskander R, Hull AD, et al. Accuracy of ultrasonography and magnetic resonance imaging in the diagnosis of placenta accreta. Obstet Gynecol 2006;108:573–81.

25. Dwyer BK, Belogolovkin V, Tran L, et al. Prenatal diagnosis of placenta accreta: sonography or magnetic resonance imaging? J Ultrasound Med 2008;27:1275–81.

26. Eller AG, Porter TF, Silver RM. Optimal management strategies for placenta accreta. BJOG 2009;116:648–54.

27. Warshak CR, Ramos GA, Eskander R, et al. Effect of predelivery diagnosis in 99 consecutive cases of placenta accreta. Obstet Gynecol 2010;115:65–9.

28. Bodner LJ, Nosher JL, Bribbin C, et al. Balloon-assisted occlusion of the internal iliac arteries in patients with placenta accreta/percreta. Cardiovasc Intervent Radiol 2006;29:354–61.

29. Shih JC, Lir KL, Shyu MK. Temporary balloon occlusion of the common iliac artery: new approach to bleeding control during cesarean hysterectomy for placenta percreta. Am J Obstet Gynecol 2005;193:1756–8.

30. Angstmann T, Gard G, Harrington T, et al. Surgical management of placenta accreta; a cohort series and suggested approach. Am J Obstet Gynecol 2010;202:38.e1–9.

31. Robinson BK, Grobman WA. Effectiveness of timing strategies for delivery of individuals with placenta previa and accreta. Obstet Gynecol 2010;116:835–42.

32. Escobar GJ, Reese HC, Greene JD. Short-term outcomes of infants born at 35 and 36 weeks gestation: we need to ask more questions. Semin Perinatol 2006;30:28–33.

33. McLaurin KK, Hall CB, Jackson EA, et al. Persistence of morbidity and cost differences between late-preterm and term infants during the first year of life. Pediatrics 2009;123:653–9.

34. MacBird T, Bronstein JM, Hall RW, et al. Late preterm infants: birth outcomes and health care utilization in the first year. Pediatrics 2010;126:e311–9.

35. Mychalishka GB, Bealor JF, Graf JL, et al. Operating on placental support: the ex utero intrapartum treatment (EXIT) procedure. J Pediatr Surg 1997;32:22–30.

36. Hedrick MH, Flake AW, Crombleholme TM, et al. The ex utero intrapartum therapy for high-risk fetal lung lesions. J Pediatr Surg 2005;40:1038–44.

37. Kunisaki SM, Barnewolt CE, Estroff JA, et al. Ex utero intrapartum treatment with extracorporeal membrane oxygenation for severe congenital diaphragmatic hernia. J Pediatr Surg 2007;42: 98–104.

38. Hedrick HL. Ex utero intrapartum therapy. Semin Pediatr Surg 2003;10:190–5.

39. Bouchard S, Johnson MP, Flake AW, et al. The EXIT procedure: experience and outcome in 31 cases. J Pediatr Surg 2002;37:418–26.

40. Morris LM, Lim FY, Elluru RG, et al. Severe micrognathia: indications for EXIT-to-airway. Fetal Diagn Ther 2009;26:162–6.

41. Costello BJ, Hueser T, Mandell D, et al. Syndromic micrognathia and peri-natal management with the ex-utero intra-partum treatment (EXIT) procedure. J Oral Maxillofac Surg 2010;39:725–8.

42. Bond SJ, Harrison MR, Slotnick RN, et al. Cesarean delivery and hysterotomy using an absorbable stapling device. Obstet Gynecol 1989;74:25–8.

43. Hirose S, Farmer DL, Lee H, et al. The ex utero intrapartum treatment procedure: looking back at the EXIT. J Pediatr Surg 2004;39:375–80.

44. Noah MM, Norton ME, Sandberg P, et al. Short-term maternal outcomes that are associated with the EXIT procedure, as compared with cesarean delivery. Am J Obstet Gynecol 2002;186:773–7.

45. Wagner W, Harrison MR. Fetal operations in the head and neck area: current state. Head Neck 2002;24:482–90.